Dr Charles Clark initially became involved in research into diabetes as a medical student almost 30 years ago, and has continued his researches since then. As a junior hospital doctor, he was awarded several research fellowships, including the prestigious R D Lawrence Research Fellowship from the British Diabetic Association (now Diabetes UK). Dr Clark was appointed the youngest Consultant Surgeon in the UK in 1988 and was subsequently appointed to Professorial level in 1991. The only medical practitioner to have been awarded three Doctorates (in Medicine, Surgery and Science), his research has been published in over 70 scientific papers in medical journals throughout the world and has encompassed all of the major complications of diabetes: eye disease; kidney disease; nerve damage; and obesity.

Maureen Clark was engaged in scientific research before becoming a professional author on diet and nutrition. Charles and Maureen's first joint venture in 2002 – *The New High Protein Diet* – became an instant bestseller, followed by a further six successful books in the series.

Dr Clark's practice is at:
14 Devonshire Place
London W1G 6HX
Tel: 020 7935 0640

Website: www.charlesvclark.com

The

DIABETES
REVOLUTION

DR CHARLES CLARK

BSc, MB ChB, DSc, MD, ChM, LLM, FRCS, FRCOphth, FRACS,
FRANZCO, FAAO, FIBiol, FAIBiol, FRMS, FSAScot, CBiol

and MAUREEN CLARK

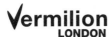
Vermilion
LONDON

9 10 8

Published in 2008 by Vermilion, an imprint of Ebury Publishing

A Random House Group company

The Random House Group Limited Reg. No. 954009

Addresses for companies within the Random House Group can be found at
www.randomhouse.co.uk

A CIP catalogue record for this book is available from the British Library

The Random House Group Limited supports The Forest Stewardship
Council (FSC), the leading international forest certification organisation.
All our titles that are printed on Greenpeace approved FSC certified paper
carry the FSC logo. Our paper procurement policy can be found at
www.rbooks.co.uk/environment

Printed and bound in the UK by
CPI Mackays, Chatham ME5 8TD

ISBN 9780091912642

Copies are available at special rates for bulk orders. Contact the sales
development team on 020 7840 8487 for more information.

To buy books by your favourite authors and register for offers, visit
www.rbooks.co.uk

The information in this book has been compiled by way of general guidance in
relation to the specific subjects addressed, but is not a substitute and not to
be relied on for medical, healthcare, pharmaceutical or other professional
advice on specific circumstances and in specific locations. Please consult
your GP before changing, stopping or starting any medical treatment. So far
as the authors are aware the information given is correct and up to date as at
March 2008. Practice, laws and regulations all change, and the reader should
obtain up to date professional advice on any such issues. The authors and
publishers disclaim, as far as the law allows, any liability arising directly or
indirectly from the use, or misuse, of the information contained in this book.

Contents

Acknowledgements

Once again, for the eighth time, we thank our children, David and Heather, whose constructive (and sometimes not so constructive) comments have evolved the recipes into their final format. Their acerbity has not diminished with age.

We thank Sian, Lady Biddulph for invaluable assistance in the preparation of the manuscript, and Hew Lorimer for producing such wonderful illustrations to explain difficult medical concepts in a unique and effective style.

Finally, we would like to thank our long-suffering editor, Julia Kellaway, for her patience with our constant revisions and her strenuous efforts to ensure such an excellent final presentation of a very important medical subject.

The Diabetes Revolution – Icon Key

 Insulin levels

 Insulin resistance

 Stress

 Drugs

 Insulin injection

 Blood pressure

 Fat cells

 Protein

 Blood sugar

 Blood

 Cholesterol

 Glucose levels

 Heart disease

 Kidney problems

 Liver problems

 Vascular disease

 Tendons

 Bones

 Visual problems

 Muscle

 Nerve sheaths

 Hardening of arteries

 Skin wrinkling

 Digestive juices

 Carbohydrates

 Hunger

 Consumption of food

 Bread

 Pasta

 Rice

 Cell membranes

 Vitamin D

 Hormones

 Viral infection

 Genetic

 Obesity

Introduction

Diabetes is a complex condition. The development of new diabetic medications, human insulin and statins have transformed the ability to control diabetes medically, but the basis of diabetic control remains diet and lifestyle. Without addressing this aspect initially, increasing levels of medication are required to control blood sugar and cholesterol, with the attendant risks of adverse side effects associated with drugs.

This programme is designed to improve the control of diabetes naturally; reducing the requirement for medication (both oral and insulin), reducing blood sugar levels, reducing cholesterol levels (and the need for statins), reducing obesity, and thereby significantly reducing the cardiovascular risk associated with diabetes. It works!

The Diabetes Revolution is for diabetic patients who would like better control of their condition, a lower risk of heart disease and a higher quality of life. These are extravagant claims but we intend to demonstrate how you can achieve these goals by diet alone – quickly, easily and permanently.

THE DIABETES EPIDEMIC

Diabetes is assuming epidemic proportions worldwide. At least 3–6 per cent of the UK population has been diagnosed; this figure rises to 10–20 per cent of people over the age of 65 years. However, this is only patients with known diabetes. The number of undiagnosed cases – particularly of type 2 diabetes – is not known but is certain to be considerably higher.

A potentially very serious disease, diabetes has major effects on quality of life – and ultimately the length of life. It is the commonest cause of blindness in those aged 18–65 years and is a major factor in the development of kidney failure, heart disease and strokes. Although genetics – the DNA which we inherit from our parents – is an important reason for many patients to develop the disease, by far the main cause of diabetes today is lifestyle – primarily diet.

DIET AND LIFESTYLE

The obvious remedy is to reverse the trend by improving diet and lifestyle.

Lifestyle changes are relatively simple:
- Stop smoking.
- Take regular exercise.
- Drink alcohol in moderation, or preferably not at all.
- Reduce dietary salt intake.

Dietary advice is much more difficult because there are so many different diabetic diets available, often with conflicting advice. While diet is not a substitute for effective medication it is the single most important factor in the control of diabetes, a fact that is often overlooked in the treatment of the disease. The correct diet leads to better control and less medication, which in turn increases quality of life and reduces the risk of drug side-effects.

Although diabetes can be controlled by drugs, these are far less effective without an appropriate diet. In fact, the wrong diet can make the disease much worse and the requirement for drugs much higher. This book will show you how to achieve the best possible control of diabetes by diet.

THE AIMS OF THIS BOOK

This book has two aims:

1. To show patients with established diabetes how to control the condition far more effectively with a dedicated dietary programme.
2. To prevent diabetes developing in patients who are at high risk, especially overweight people.

How effective is the programme? Very. In our clinic, we are able to reduce the amount of insulin required by a type 1 diabetic (see page 7) by an average of 30–40 per cent within two weeks of commencing the programme. All type 2 diabetics have reported significant reduction in their requirement of oral medication, and many early-stage type 2 diabetics (see page 1) have managed to achieve acceptable control of blood sugar levels without medication.

WHY OUR SYSTEM IS DIFFERENT

The basis of diabetes management is good control but this can sometimes be difficult to achieve, no matter how hard you try to keep to the instructions on the diet you have been advised to follow. And, as blood sugar increases, more and more medication is required to control it.

But this need not be the case. The Diabetes Revolution has been developed to improve control of diabetes by lowering blood sugar levels naturally. How can we be so sure it works? Because it is based on strict medical principles: the results of the measurement of insulin and blood sugar. In other words, it is based on solid, objective medical facts.

These are bold claims, but true! See for yourself the levels of success our diet has achieved by reading the case histories from diabetic patients in Chapters 6 and 7; you will probably recognise similarities to your own situation.

This is not a textbook; it is not designed to teach you all of the medical intricacies of diabetes. It is a description of a medically based dietary programme specifically developed to be as simple to understand and follow as possible, and which will dramatically improve your control of diabetes.

Our programme is in two stages. During the initial stage, the aim is to get your blood sugar levels under control. Once you have achieved that, you can move on to the maintenance phase, which allows you to introduce a wider variety of foods.

Chapter 1   What is Diabetes?

There are two main types of diabetes: type 2 and type 1.

Type 2 Diabetes

Type 2 diabetes is by far the most common form of the disease, affecting up to 90 per cent of all diabetic patients, mostly people aged over 40. It is also known as non-insulin-dependent diabetes. People with type 2 diabetes are either unable to make enough of the hormone insulin or cannot use insulin effectively. Our bodies need insulin to move the glucose (or sugar) we get from food out of the bloodstream and into the cells of the body. This type of diabetes tends to run in families. The risk also increases with age and obesity (particularly fat stored around the abdomen).

Sometimes people develop the disease without knowing it and have few symptoms. Others experience excessive thirst and urination, constipation, infections, blurred vision and tingling in the hands and feet. Your doctor can diagnose or rule out type 2 diabetes through urine and blood glucose tests.

INSULIN RESISTANCE

Eating starchy carbohydrates stimulates the pancreas to produce insulin. Refined carbohydrates are simple sugars that quickly raise levels of glucose in the body. These can be found, for example, in white bread and sugary foods. The more refined carbohydrates you eat, the more insulin you need to inject (in type 1 diabetes) or the higher the level of insulin produced by your body (in type 2 diabetes).

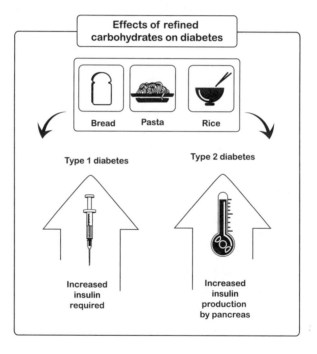

Problems start to arise when the body makes too much insulin. Every single cell in the body requires some insulin, which is essential for the cell to utilise (metabolise) carbohydrates, fats and proteins. Every cell has receptors to allow it to absorb insulin.

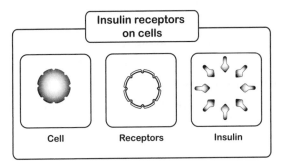

Each cell can only take in so much insulin before it stops absorbing it. The receptors become 'blunted' and decrease in number, leading to 'insulin resistance'.

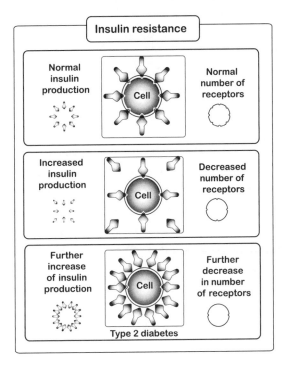

Essentially, a vicious circle develops: the more insulin we make, the fewer receptors we have on our cells, and therefore the more insulin we have to make in response. This vicious circle continues until eventually the pancreas cannot make any more insulin.

The other main function of insulin is to control the level of sugar in the blood.

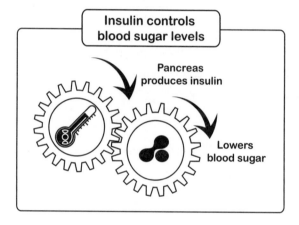

Refined carbohydrates stimulate increased insulin production (in type 2 diabetes) or increased requirement for insulin (in type 1 diabetes). This causes insulin resistance with reduced numbers of insulin receptors on every cell of the body, which in turn causes increased levels of insulin, either from the pancreas (type 2) or by injection (type 1).

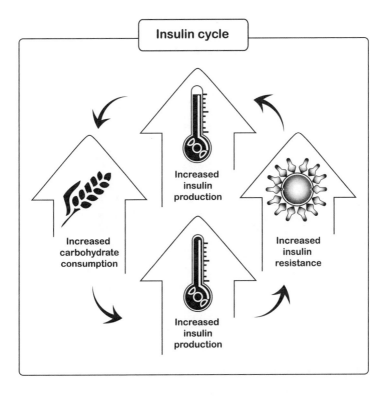

Eventually, the insulin resistance produced by the cells of the body means that we cannot produce any more insulin to control the sugar. The sugar level starts to rise, and this is the point at which we make the diagnosis of type 2 diabetes.

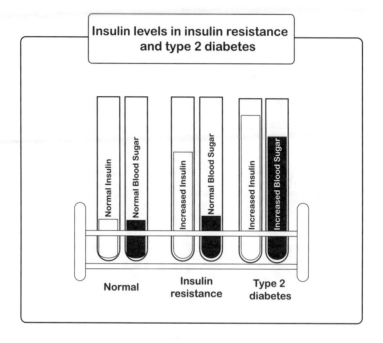

High levels of insulin can also lead to a condition called 'metabolic syndrome', which can be a precursor to type 2 diabetes. The characteristic features of this condition are:

- elevated insulin levels
- raised blood pressure
- obesity
- elevated triglyceride levels (fats in the blood leading to heart disease)

Although diabetes may be diagnosed on the basis of blood sugar, insulin levels are elevated for a considerable period – perhaps many years – before the disease develops. This is known as the 'pre-diabetic stage'. This also explains why type 2 diabetes involves high levels of insulin, which are still insufficient to control the blood sugar.

A high level of insulin has potentially serious side effects, including the elevated risk of heart disease due to insulin:

■ increasing hardening of the arteries
■ increasing LDL (bad) cholesterol
■ increasing triglycerides in the blood
■ reducing protective HDL cholesterol
■ increasing the production of fat cells
■ reducing the facility to burn fat cells

The raised levels of insulin in type 2 diabetes actually cause the patient to increase weight and produce more fat. For more on insulin, see page 9.

Type 1 Diabetes

Also known as insulin-dependent diabetes, type 1 diabetes affects 3–25 per cent of all diabetic patients and occurs primarily in people under 40, including children. People with type 1 diabetes produce insufficient insulin; some patients may produce no insulin. The disease may be inherited or caused by factors in the environment. In simple terms this means either that you were programmed genetically to develop the disease, or that something in your environment caused the condition – of which the most common cause is a viral infection.

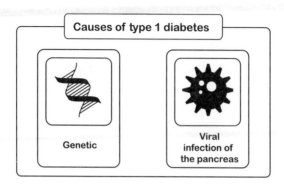

People with type 1 diabetes tend to be slim, sometimes even thin. Before being diagnosed, they will feel ill for a few weeks and experience symptoms such as severe thirst, frequent urination and weight loss. They need to be given insulin quickly to prevent a rapid deterioration of their condition. Insulin must be replaced by injection on a frequent basis during the day.

The Diabetes Revolution is particularly effective in type 1 diabetic patients with reasonably stable control* for the following reasons:

1. The more refined carbohydrates in your diet, the more insulin you need to inject.
2. The more insulin, the more potential complications from insulin.
3. The logical conclusion is that reducing refined carbohydrates in your diet will lower your insulin requirement and reduce life-threatening complications.

* The diet is not suitable for brittle diabetics or diabetics with very variable control as this must be monitored exclusively by a hospital diabetic department.

On this programme, the majority of patients experience significantly reduced requirements for insulin almost immediately, in many cases a reduction of up to 40 per cent within two weeks. This is an incredible improvement in diabetic control in a very short period.

This system is so effective in controlling diabetes that you have to introduce it gradually into your daily programme to prevent hypoglycaemia. If the level of blood glucose is rapidly reducing as a result of the diet, it is essential to monitor blood glucose measurements four or five times every day and adjust insulin accordingly.

Insulin – the Key to Diabetic Control

The hormone insulin is the key to diabetic control. But the *amount* of insulin produced is totally different in type 1 and type 2 diabetes:

- In type 1 diabetes, the patient produces very little insulin.
- In most type 2 diabetics, the patient has a high level of insulin.

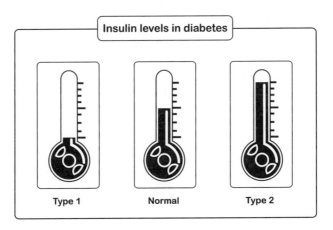

Insulin levels in diabetes

| Type 1 | Normal | Type 2 |

Can this be possible? How can these opposite levels of insulin produce similar symptoms? Very easily! The answer is that in both types of diabetes the patient is not making enough insulin for their needs.

- In type 1 diabetes the patient has insufficient insulin and therefore requires additional insulin by injection.
- In type 2 diabetes, the patient has a high level of insulin but it is still not enough due to insulin resistance (see page 2), and therefore requires supplementation with medication and eventually insulin injections.

DIET AND INSULIN PRODUCTION

What stimulates the pancreas to produce insulin? There are many factors including stress and certain medications.

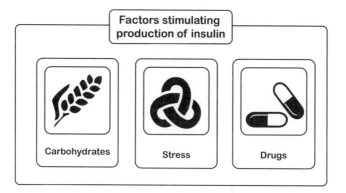

However, the single most important stimulus for insulin production is food. Production of insulin is stimulated by carbohydrates in our diet and, to a much lesser degree, by protein. It is not stimulated by dietary fat.

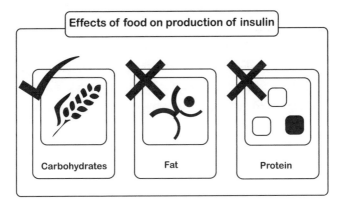

Although insulin per se is not bad – in fact, a certain amount of insulin is absolutely essential for health – the problem is that our modern diet stimulates the production of far too much insulin.

The Problem with Excess Insulin

First, insulin causes excess calories to be stored as fat. Even worse, it actually prevents the breakdown of fat cells, so your body is unable to use your stored fat as energy.

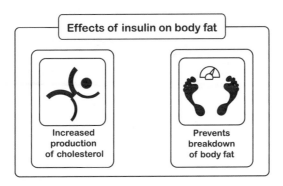

Other, even more negative, effects on health of excess insulin include:

- Excess production of cholesterol by the liver, causing raised cholesterol levels and increasing the risk of heart disease.
- Stimulating the kidneys to retain excess water and salt, which can lead to raised blood pressure.
- Increasing the muscular component of the artery walls, further contributing to high blood pressure.
- Increasing the levels of fats in the blood called 'triglycerides', a very significant indicator of heart disease.

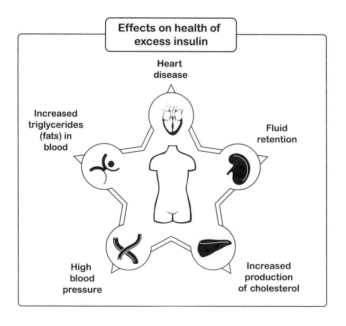

Effects on health of excess insulin

Heart disease

Increased triglycerides (fats) in blood

Fluid retention

High blood pressure

Increased production of cholesterol

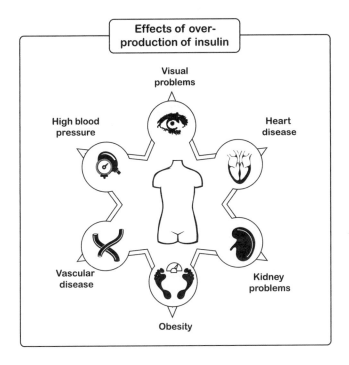

Insulin levels cannot be lowered by medication. They can be reduced only by altering the diet. This is common sense as, in the majority of patients, the problem is caused by excess carbohydrates. The obvious solution is to reduce the amount of refined carbohydrates we eat. The next chapter looks at how you can start to take practical steps to reduce your insulin levels through your diet.

TO SUMMARISE THE PROBLEM:

- Insulin is a hormone which affects every cell in the body.
- Insulin is absolutely essential for health but too much insulin is detrimental to health.
- Refined carbohydrates are the main stimulus for insulin production.
- Too much refined carbohydrate in the diet causes the production of too much insulin.

And the consequences of overproduction of insulin (insulinaemia) are increased risk of:

- obesity
- heart disease
- high blood pressure
- arthritis (due to obesity)
- diabetes
- kidney failure (secondary to diabetes)
- visual problems (possibly leading to blindness) as a result of diabetes

Chapter 2 Controlling Diabetes through Diet

There are so many seemingly conflicting diets proposed in the management of diabetes that one may reasonably question whether there really is a single, effective diet. There are high-carb and low-carb diets, low-fat and low-calorie diets, high-protein diets, GI diets, GL diets... No wonder both the patient and the medical profession can be totally confused – however, the evidence clearly points in one direction.

GI Diets

The most effective diet for diabetes control is one based on consuming foods with a low glycaemic index (GI). These are often referred to as GI diets. The glycaemic index measures the effect of food on raising blood sugar levels. Foods that score low on the GI are the building blocks of this dietary approach.

GI diets have been demonstrated to lower insulin levels, reduce blood glucose, reduce the 'bad' blood fats (triglycerides and low density lipoproteins) and increase the 'good' blood fats (high density lipoproteins). Unfortunately, there are several different GI diets currently available, some definitely more effective than others. To add to the confusion, a GI diet can be both low-carb (as it is lower in *refined* carbohydrates such as bread, rice and pasta) and high-carb at the same time (as it is high in *unrefined* carbohydrates by incorporating almost unlimited vegetables).

The effects of a properly managed GI diet are:

- more stable glucose levels
- lower insulin resistance in patients with type 2 diabetes and metabolic syndrome (and therefore reduced requirement for oral medication)
- reduced requirement for insulin in a type 1 diabetic
- reduction of serum triglycerides and increase in high density lipoproteins, significantly reducing cardiovascular risk

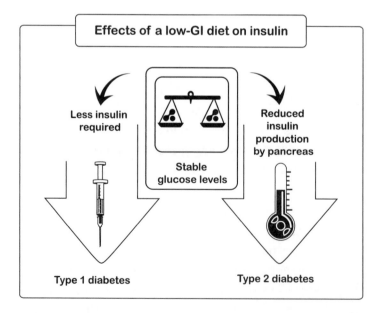

Effects of a low-GI diet on insulin

Less insulin required

Reduced insulin production by pancreas

Stable glucose levels

Type 1 diabetes

Type 2 diabetes

In general, high carb equals high GI. However, some low-GI foods are definitely not healthy in excess. For example, pure fat has a GI of zero but we would certainly not advocate this in your programme. It is important to emphasise that a GI diet which is low in refined carbohydrates is *not* a high-fat diet. It merely includes natural fats in moderation (such as extra-virgin olive oil, cheese, eggs, fatty fish). Foods incorporating trans fats (the really bad fats) are still excluded.

Similarly, a GI diet is not the same as a low-carb diet. Both restrict high-GI foods such as bread, pasta and rice, but some low-carb diets also restrict the unrefined carbohydrates in vegetables, which is intrinsically dangerous. The problem is not the reduction in carbohydrates per se but rather the vitamin and mineral deficiencies that inevitably result from such a restricted diet unless comprehensive vitamin and mineral supplementation is rigorously implemented. A diet with virtually unrestricted vegetables does not have this problem.

There are numerous studies proving the ineffectiveness of a low-fat/high-carbohydrate diet on blood fats. The diets that were successful in improving the lipid profile in these studies were all based on the low-GI principle, replacing refined carbohydrates with unrefined carbohydrates, proteins and fats.

HOW GI DIETS AFFECT INSULIN

Insulin is the key to effective management of type 2 diabetes because it controls levels of blood sugar and blood fat. A GI diet lowers insulin resistance relatively quickly, within 10–14 days. As insulin is the hormone controlling deposition of body fat, lowering insulin levels has the additional advantage of healthy weight loss.

The measurement of insulin and cholesterol levels makes the task of controlling diabetes much easier. Success is apparent as the patient loses weight and, more importantly, this is associated with the lowering of blood glucose and cholesterol. This is clearly demonstrated by a typical case study of a 54-year-old male type 2 diabetic patient. After one month on the GI programme, these were his results:

- a reduction of fasting serum insulin by 44 per cent
- a reduction of fasting triglycerides ('bad' fats) by 55 per cent
- a reduction of LDL (more 'bad' fats) by 30 per cent
- an increase in HDL ('good' fats) by 15 per cent
- a reduction of total cholesterol by 32 per cent
- a reduction of weight by 2 kg

The Diabetes Revolution in Practice

You are more likely to continue with a diet if you see results quickly. If you experience weight loss combined with improved diabetic control within a short period (less than two weeks), this acts as a powerful incentive to continue, especially if you feel better and have more energy and less fluctuation of blood glucose. After years of struggling with weight loss and glucose stability, patients on the diet begin to feel in control for the first time.

The Diabetes Revolution is a revolutionary programme

because it completely reverses a number of previous theories. For example, a diet based on refined carbohydrates (such as bread and rice) will raise cholesterol levels, whereas a diet that includes eggs and cheese can actually lower cholesterol levels. The diet has been developed over many years and adapted according to the results of blood tests on patients, so it is based on medical facts, not conjecture. There are two phases that are quite different: the initial phase and the maintenance phase. Foods excluded in the initial phase are reintroduced later, making this a dynamic diet, not one that is fixed or rigid.

The underlying principle of the programme is the unrestricted inclusion of healthy, nutritious foods and the exclusion of unhealthy foods. This means that all of the essential proteins, fats, vitamins and minerals are present in abundance and the diet is therefore *naturally* balanced. However, the definition of 'healthy' and 'unhealthy' differs from other programmes. Our results have conclusively demonstrated that refined carbohydrates (such as bread, pasta and rice) are very unhealthy for diabetics, raising blood glucose and cholesterol levels. So, this programme is not only different from other GI diets in practice, it is **the only diabetic dietary programme to substantiate its claims by results of blood glucose, cholesterol and insulin measurements**.

Manipulating the glycaemic index is the key to controlling diabetes and reducing coronary heart disease. It is simple, effective and inexpensive. Replacing refined carbohydrates with unrefined carbohydrates in the diet will lower insulin and glucose levels. Of course, achieving the full advantage of a GI programme is not this simple but these easy steps will produce quick results and convince both the doctor and the patient of its effectiveness.

The diet changes as diabetic control improves. Refined carbohydrates can be reintroduced in a controlled and scientific manner in the maintenance phase of the programme. For example, although both have the same carbohydrate content, arborio rice has a much lower glycaemic index (and capacity to stimulate insulin production) than jasmine rice and is therefore more suitable to a diabetic diet.

THE DIET AND TYPE 1 DIABETES

Although it is safe to introduce this diet in patients with metabolic syndrome and type 2 diabetes – measuring glucose regularly to reduce oral medication appropriately – extreme caution must be exercised in the case of type 1 diabetics. If the patient transfers from a typical high-carb diet to a GI programme, blood glucose must be measured very regularly and insulin reduced accordingly as the requirement for insulin can reduce significantly in a relatively short period. Reductions of 50 per cent are not uncommon. The patient must therefore be warned to reduce insulin and the doctor should monitor the situation closely to prevent hypoglycaemia.

THE CARBOHYDRATE CYCLE

To achieve optimal control of diabetes you need to reduce your refined carbohydrate intake to approximately 60 grams per day. Tables of carbohydrate content are given in the Appendix (page 262), and there are some general guidelines below. For example, one slice of bread contains 15–17 grams of carbohydrate and an egg contains none.

To appreciate the central role of insulin in diabetes you have to understand the role of carbohydrates in the control of diabetes: the carbohydrate cycle.

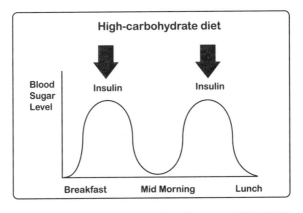

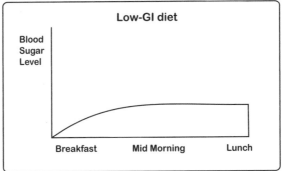

Carbohydrates are – in simple terms – sugars and starches. They are absorbed from the digestive tract reasonably quickly, which is the reason why we get a rapid energy boost from a bar of chocolate or a pastry. But – and this is the important part – when our blood sugar levels go up, it stimulates insulin to be released, which then starts to lower the blood sugar level very quickly. The sugar level in the blood goes down rapidly (hypoglycaemia); we feel weak and faint so we have another sweet food to boost our sugar level. Once again, we feel better for a while, then insulin kicks in to lower our blood sugar and make us feel weak.

So the cycle begins again. All carbohydrates are ultimately broken down to simple sugars. Some carbohydrates are complex (such as potato); some are simple (such as glucose). However, complex carbohydrates are not necessarily healthier for diabetics than simple carbohydrates!

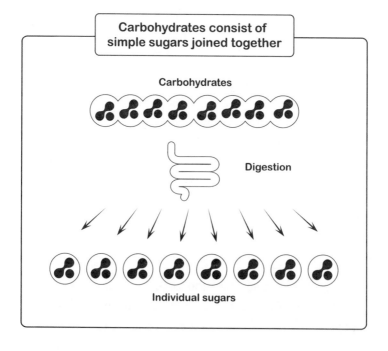

Carbohydrates consist of simple sugars joined together

Carbohydrates

Digestion

Individual sugars

Incredible though it may seem, when you consume a potato, your blood sugar level rises at *exactly the same rate as pure sugar*. Potatoes and sugar have the same glycaemic index of 100 (see overleaf). So simply including complex carbohydrates in your diet does not prevent the problem of increasing blood sugar levels stimulating an increase in the body's requirement for insulin. This doesn't mean that complex carbohydrates aren't healthier than simple carbohydrates – of course they are – but there is more to the control of diabetes than replacing simple carbs with complex carbs. Your body simply can't cope with too much sugar in the diet.

The problem is that it is not always easy to see how many carbohydrates are in everyday foods. Remember, carbohydrates are simply sugars joined together. It is amazing how much sugar is 'hidden' in many foods. The impact of the statement becomes obvious when you realise the number of teaspoons of sugar present in 100 g of common foods.

Did you realise that a typical serving of pasta or rice (100 g or 4 oz) is converted to 12–14 teaspoons of sugar in your body? Or that a banana is the equivalent to seven teaspoons of sugar? Although natural sugars (such as those found in fruit) are much healthier than white sugar, your body cannot differentiate between them. The more refined carbohydrates you consume, the more sugar you are effectively consuming, and the more insulin you will require – either by injection or from the pancreas.

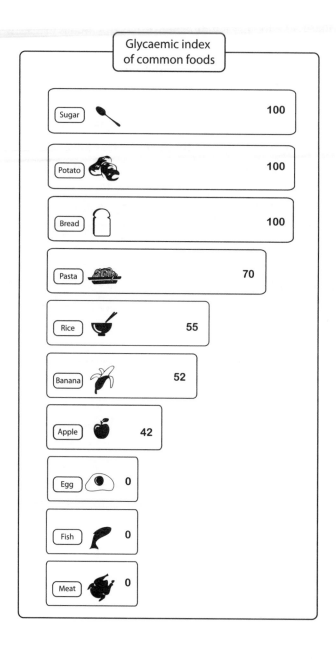

Glycaemic index of common foods

Sugar — 100

Potato — 100

Bread — 100

Pasta — 70

Rice — 55

Banana — 52

Apple — 42

Egg — 0

Fish — 0

Meat — 0

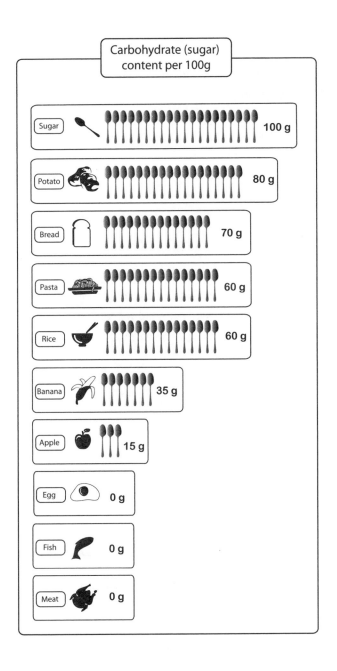

Carbohydrate (sugar)
content per 100g

Sugar   100 g

Potato   80 g

Bread   70 g

Pasta   60 g

Rice   60 g

Banana   35 g

Apple   15 g

Egg   0 g

Fish   0 g

Meat   0 g

Every diabetic has probably experienced the constant roller coaster of energy levels. Even worse are the difficult mood swings that accompany the energy fluctuations.

To summarise:

- When we are hungry, we eat carbohydrates, which provide a rapid source of energy.
- This stimulates the production of insulin by the body, which quickly lowers the blood sugar, making us feel weak and irritable, so we have more carbohydrates to make us feel better – but only briefly.
- Insulin then caps its performance by stimulating the deposit of excess carbohydrate as fat, especially around the waist and hips. Even worse, insulin actually prevents body fat being used to provide energy, so we can never break down body fat if insulin levels are elevated.

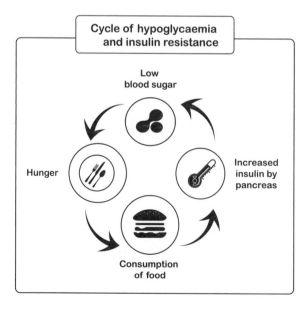

Cycle of hypoglycaemia and insulin resistance

Low blood sugar

Increased insulin by pancreas

Consumption of food

Hunger

This problem of constant fluctuations in blood glucose can only be solved by reducing the levels of insulin.

- In type 1 diabetes, this means reducing the *requirement* for insulin by injection.
- In type 2 diabetes, the significantly elevated levels of insulin need to be lowered.

If we reduce the insulin, hypoglycaemia doesn't occur so we don't become weak and irritable and we don't feel the need to eat more carbohydrate for energy. And we don't make fat to be deposited on our waists and hips.

Even better, if we lower insulin levels, the body mechanisms are actually directed to burn body fat preferentially. But how can you reduce your requirement for insulin? Once again, the answer is very simple:

Reduce your intake of refined carbohydrates

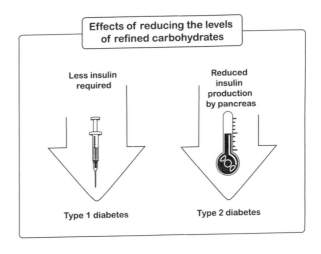

The production of insulin is not significantly stimulated by fats or proteins, so if you cut down drastically on refined carbohydrates, your requirement for insulin levels reduces naturally.

Many diabetic diets instruct you to increase your daily intake of carbohydrates, usually as cereals, grains, pasta and rice. So you weren't a failure after all, it just wasn't medically possible to achieve good control of diabetes on a diet based on refined carbohydrates.

Our bodies do not need, and were never designed to cope with, large quantities of refined carbohydrates such as the immense loads of refined sugars and starches in the pre-packaged foods which form the basis of the modern Western diet. If we cut out the foods which our bodies cannot safely tolerate, insulin production returns to a more 'normal' level in type 2 diabetes, and the need for insulin by injection is significantly reduced in type 1 diabetes.

REFINED AND UNREFINED CARBOHYDRATES

There are two distinct forms of carbohydrate in health terms:

- **Unrefined** 'natural' carbohydrates (such as vegetables, salads and fruit).
- **Refined** 'processed' carbohydrates (such as white bread, pasta, rice, pre-packaged foods, cakes and confectionery).

In the diet, vegetables and salads are included virtually without restriction, and fruit can be consumed in moderation. Refined carbohydrates, on the other hand, are almost completely excluded.

The differences between 'healthy' unrefined carbo-hydrates and 'unhealthy' refined carbohydrates will be discussed in the next chapter. However, in simple terms foods may be categorised as follows:

Foods Containing No Refined Carbohydrates

- animal-based products, including beef, pork, lamb and poultry
- fish and shellfish
- eggs
- cheese
- vegetables
- fruit
- dairy products (milk, yoghurt, cream)
- fruit juices
- pulses (peas, beans, lentils)
- all 'pure' fats, including oils (such as olive oil) and butter
- herbs
- spices
- low-calorie soft drinks
- tea
- artificial sweeteners

Foods Based on Refined Carbohydrates

- bread
- rice
- pasta
- most pre-packaged savoury foods
- all cakes, confectionery, sweets and biscuits
- all pies and pastries
- flour
- all cereals (including breakfast cereals)
- beer/cider/sweet white wine/fortified wines (sherry, port)

REDUCING YOUR INTAKE OF REFINED CARBOHYDRATES

As we have seen, in order to reduce your requirement for insulin you need to decrease your intake of refined carbohydrates to about 60 grams per day. This is remarkably easy to achieve, without resorting to measuring or weighing food portions in the initial phase of the programme. Simply by following the guidelines in the lists on page 32 (lists of 'foods included without restriction' and 'foods to which restrictions apply'), you will have achieved this target. When you become more adventurous in the later stages of the programme, use the tables in the Appendix to guide you regarding the carbohydrate content of various food groups.

Never reduce your carbohydrate intake to less than 60 grams per day. Doing so will mean that you are restricting vegetables from your diet, which will inevitably lead to nutritional deficiencies. The only alternative is to take multivitamin supplements but, if you keep to the level of 60 grams of unrefined carbohydrates, that will not be necessary.

TAILORING THE DIET TO YOUR NEEDS

The Diabetes Revolution is not based simply on the carbohydrate content of foods. On the contrary, it takes into account many other relevant factors:

- the glycaemic index of foods
- the insulinogenic effect of some foods (see opposite)
- the fat content of food

The essential problem with providing a perfect dietary programme for every diabetic is that each individual is intrinsically unique. This seems obvious but it has very serious medical (and therefore dietary) implications. For example, one patient may have a high insulin level while another's may be lower (even though they may both have identical blood sugar levels). One individual may be grossly overweight while another may be only slightly overweight. In each and every case the response to a medically based diet will obviously be different because the individuals have different medical characteristics at the start of the diet.

Similarly, the effect carbohydrates have on stimulating insulin production does not follow the simple rules we might expect in every case. For example, in some individuals, dairy products produce a far higher insulin response than their carbohydrate content would merit. This means that the insulin response is higher than expected on the basis of the carbohydrate content alone – the insulinogenic effect.

The Role of Dietary Fat

The fat content of food must form an integral part of a balanced programme for the control of diabetes. Contrary to popular belief, not all fats are detrimental to health. Some are, but probably not the ones you expect. In fact, some fats are actually healthy and will help to control diabetes.

Let's put the fat myth into perspective. We need certain fats for life: to build cell walls, sheaths around nerve cells and hormones (chemical messengers in the body), to name just a few essential roles for fats in the body. However, we need 'healthy' fats (described in Chapter 3), not the 'unhealthy' trans fats present in many pre-packaged foods and cakes.

Principles of the Programme

In general, the following is a simple guide to foods *included* or *excluded* from the diet:

Foods included without restriction
- fish and shellfish
- herbs and spices
- lean meat
- poultry
- most vegetables (except those with a high-carbohydrate content, such as potatoes and parsnips)
- salads (but restrict tomatoes to three per day initially)
- low-calorie soft drinks
- tea
- artificial sweeteners

Foods to which restrictions apply
- dairy products (restrict milk to tea and coffee only in the first month; natural yoghurt **only** in the first month, to a maximum of three 150 ml portions per week)
- oils and dressings (in moderation)
- eggs (maximum of six per week)
- fruit (restricted to one piece per day for the first month, increasing to three pieces in maintenance phase. One piece could be a bowl of berries, perhaps with natural yoghurt. Bananas, mangoes and pineapple are **absolutely prohibited** in the first month as these fruits are high in sugar)
- nuts (50 grams per day, especially brazil nuts, hazelnuts, almonds and walnuts. Pistachios, peanuts and cashew nuts are **absolutely prohibited** in the first two months)

- sauces (if high sugar content)
- pulses (up to 50 grams per day)
- cheese (up to 50 grams per day – but no crackers or oatcakes)

Foods excluded during the initial phase

- pasta, rice, flour, grains and cereals (pasta and rice are excluded during the initial phase as these foods are very high in refined carbohydrates, up to 73 per cent. Bread is restricted to a maximum of one slice per day in the initial phase. However, all these foods are reintroduced in the maintenance phase, page 227)
- biscuits, cakes and pastries
- desserts and sugars
- all full-sugar drinks, such as lemonade, colas, energy drinks
- fruit juice
- fast food
- snack foods
- pre-packaged savoury foods
- chocolate and sweets
- potatoes and parsnips
- bananas, mangoes and pineapple
- jasmine rice (very high GI)

ALCOHOL

In diabetes, alcohol intake must be restricted for many medical reasons.

For the first month of the programme, alcohol is prohibited. In the maintenance phase, alcohol can be included to the following maximum amounts. It should be stressed that these are the absolute maximum daily intake, not recommended amounts:

- alcoholic spirits (whisky, gin, brandy) – maximum of two measures per day, or
- red wine – maximum of two 175 ml glasses per day, or
- dry white wine – maximum of two 175 ml glasses per day

The following alcoholic drinks should be permanently excluded (apart from special occasions) as they are very high in sugar content and will seriously disrupt effective control of diabetes:

- beer, lager, cider, sweet white wine, champagne, sherry and port

Of course, the occasional glass of champagne at a wedding or Christmas will have no undue effect but in general these drinks should be avoided.

Chapter 3 Why the Diabetes Revolution Works

This chapter will explain why certain foods are included and others are excluded on the Diabetes Revolution – in essence, why it works – and why you can't break the rules and still be successful.

I firmly believe, as a Consultant Surgeon in practice for over 25 years, that the single most important factor in successful medical treatment is to involve the patient completely in the management of the case. In effect, this means that the patient should have full knowledge and understanding of the condition affecting them, and should fully comprehend the line of treatment and, most importantly, the reasons for it. They can then make informed decisions regarding their own health and future. After all, it is their body, and no one is going to care about it as much as they do!

In my experience, most diabetics are concerned when they don't know what's happening to them – the fear of the unknown – and have fewer worries when they understand the situation, and can be involved in solving the problem.

What has this got to do with diet? Everything! Your diet ultimately determines the control (or lack of control) of diabetes. It dictates whether you will be well or ill, and it may ultimately cause your early death. Diet is therefore the essential component part of diabetic control.

You don't have to read this chapter to successfully control diabetes. However, if you take the time to do so (and re-read it later), you will understand what you have to do – and why – and you will start to take control of your own health. Everyone has the intellectual capacity to understand the principles of nutrition when simply explained, and to take control of their own destiny thereafter.

Some of the information has been covered briefly in earlier chapters, but will be looked at in more detail here. More importantly, it will explain why you need these various components in your diet.

The Goodness in Your Food

One of the words used to describe the intrinsic qualities in foods, which has fallen from favour in recent years, is 'goodness'. This word is perfect for conveying the value – or lack of value – of the various foods in our diet. When someone tells you that a particular food is 'full of goodness', or that another food has 'no goodness in it', you immediately know exactly what they mean. Or do you? As with all excellent expressions, this term is often hijacked by advertisers as logos or catchphrases to tell you what they want you to think, rather than the truth.

A diet must be nutritionally safe – in other words, it must include all of the nutrients essential for health. Unfortunately, many diets are not safe. For example, a typical low-calorie diet requires you to consume fewer calories (as food) than you require. This inevitably means you get fewer nutrients and, unless you are very careful, you can end up malnourished.

It certainly isn't necessary for you to become an expert on nutrition, but you must be sure that you will obtain all of the essential nutrients from your diet. Interestingly, this information isn't usually given in books for diabetics, presumably because very few diets actually provide all the nutrition you need – in other words, the diets are actually making you unwell!

The Diabetes Revolution is different. While it is quite easy to obtain all the essential nutrients on a diet including foods of animal origin, it is also relatively simple to do so on a typical vegetarian diet while excluding refined carbohydrates. White rice, pasta, bread, sugars and other refined carbohydrates provide no nutrition whatsoever (unless nutrients have been added to them). They are merely sources of energy, which can be provided equally well by essential proteins and fats. Refined carbohydrates have no intrinsic vitamins or minerals; in fact, in their natural state they are so devoid of nutrients that vitamins and minerals are routinely added to them as a result of government legislation.

So that you can be absolutely certain that you are getting all the essential nutrients for health from your diet, here is a brief look at the most important elements of the Diabetes Revolution. Although it isn't possible to include all essential nutrients here, you can be certain they will be included in the diet.

PROTEINS

Proteins are the building blocks of life. Or, to be more accurate, proteins are made up of amino acids, which are the building blocks of the body. When we eat foods containing protein, our digestive system breaks down the protein into its component amino acids, and joins them together again as the structural proteins we need.

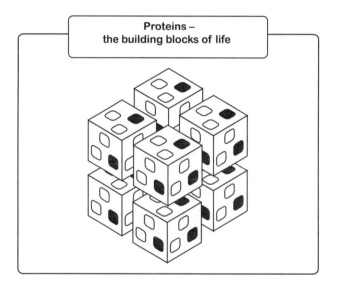

Proteins –
the building blocks of life

Proteins are essential, not only to build the structures we can see – like skin, bones, hair and nails – but also the myriad tissues that we can't see, but which keep us alive: the blood cells, immune system, nervous system, and chemicals that make reactions occur, called enzymes. This is deliberately intended to be a very simplistic view of the complexity of protein chemistry, but you can see that if you don't have the necessary building blocks, the essential structures will not be formed.

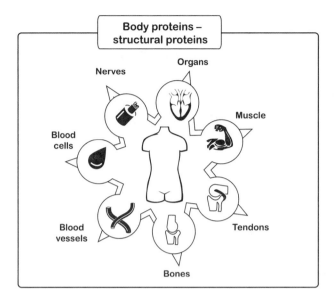

Body proteins – structural proteins

Nerves

Organs

Muscle

Blood cells

Blood vessels

Tendons

Bones

The bottom line is, we need certain proteins for life. Although all of the proteins we require can be supplied from plant sources, 'complete' proteins (which means they contain all of the essential amino acids we need) come primarily from animal sources: beef, pork, fish, poultry and eggs. Animal sources of protein will form the basis of the programme for two main reasons:

1. They supply all of the essential amino acids to prevent protein deficiencies (which are very serious).
2. It is much more complicated to ensure that you obtain all of the necessary amino acids from plants alone.

The only plant source which contains all of the essential amino acids is tofu, a soya product. It is certainly possible to follow a healthy vegetarian low-GI programme, providing eggs are included. Vitamin B12 is not present in plant foods so a supplement is necessary for vegans.

To make things even easier, animal proteins (beef, pork, fish, poultry and eggs) contain no refined carbohydrates, so they follow the rules of the programme, as protein and fats, unlike carbohydrates, do not stimulate the production of insulin.

FATS

Fats are made up of their own building blocks (called fatty acids), similar to the situation with proteins, and we need certain essential fatty acids to live. We also need some fat in our diet for correct absorption of certain nutrients (see 'Vitamins and Minerals', page 46). But all fats are not equal! Some are very good, and some are very harmful.

Essential Fatty Acids

Essential fatty acids are usually divided into two groups: omega-3 and omega-6.

Omega-3 fatty acids are found in oily fish (such as herring, mackerel, salmon, sardines and tuna), fish oils, eggs (the yolk), nuts, nut oils, and certain vegetable oils (especially flaxseed).

Omega-6 fatty acids are found in eggs (the yolk), seeds and seed oils (in particular sunflower, safflower and sesame), whole grains, certain vegetables and vegetable oils. Omega-6 fatty acids are also present in evening primrose and borage oils.

Not only do we need these essential fatty acids, but they also need to be in the correct proportion for health, which is 2:1 of omega-6 to omega-3. The typical Western diet contains large amounts of corn oil which increases this proportion to about 9:1, so although there are essential fatty acids in the diet, they are not in the correct proportions for health.

A special mention must be made of olive oil, which has a high proportion of monounsaturated oils, but is relatively low in essential fatty acids. It is incredibly healthy, not least because of its vitamin E, magnesium and antioxidant content – especially polyphenols.

So, obviously, we need to incorporate these fats into our diet. But we are not going to add them to the diet; we are going to replace certain other types of fat in the diet with these 'healthy' fats. For example, by cooking with extra-virgin olive oil, and including fish, eggs and certain vegetables in our diet, we have simultaneously created a diet high in protein, essential fatty acids, vitamins, minerals and antioxidants (see page 43), with no refined carbohydrates. Simple!

Do not misinterpret the message of this chapter. It is not intended to advocate a high-fat diet, and although you are eating 'pure' fats, you will actually be eating less fat. This is because most of the 'bad' fats are incorporated in foods with refined sugars and carbohydrates (such as cakes, pastries, pizza, pies, processed and packaged foods, 'fast' foods, potato crisps, chips) – which you have excluded from your diet. Instead, you have replaced them with essential fatty acids in eggs, fish, vegetables and nuts, among other sources.

These foods are more than just 'fats', even 'essential fats'! They contain high-quality complete proteins and essential vitamins and minerals (see page 46). They are also a major source of antioxidants, which keep us healthy, prevent cancer and various other serious medical conditions, and help to prevent ageing.

CARBOHYDRATES

Carbohydrates provide energy in our diet, and little else. 'Refined' carbohydrates provide energy in our diet and *nothing* else, apart from causing increased production of insulin which promotes fat storage. It would seem fairly obvious to the most casual observer that we don't need refined carbohydrates in our life and therefore we are going to exclude them!

However, apart from refined sugar, carbohydrates are seldom 'pure'; rather they are mixed with other constituents in various foods. Carbohydrates are present in very unhealthy foods when mixed with fats (as in chips, cakes and pizzas) and in healthy foods such as vegetables. The carbohydrates in fresh vegetables are very different from those in refined foods. In fresh vegetables, the carbohydrates are 'complex', which means they are absorbed much more slowly and evenly over a period of time, rather than the rapid absorption (and associated rapid release of insulin) that occurs with refined sugars. Much more importantly in health terms, carbohydrates in fresh vegetables are incorporated with vitamins, minerals, proteins and fibre, all of which we need for survival. They are not associated with refined fats, only with essential fatty acids (in some vegetables).

A successful diet to control diabetes involves reducing intake of 'bad' carbohydrates: the refined carbohydrates present in cakes, confectionery, chocolate and sweets, as well as bread products, pasta and rice. By avoiding these refined carbohydrates, you simultaneously reduce your fat intake dramatically, because most trans fats are incorporated in foods with refined carbohydrates.

FREE RADICALS AND ANTIOXIDANTS

'Free radicals' and 'antioxidants' are probably the most important factors in preventing diseases and ageing. In each of our cells (of which we have billions), thousands of chemical reactions occur every second. To release the energy from our food, the chemical reactions produce 'free radicals', which are essentially molecules that have lost an electron.

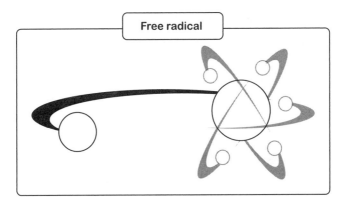

Their natural reaction is to try to take an electron from another molecule, which causes damage to the cells of our body – especially as this process occurs millions of times per second!

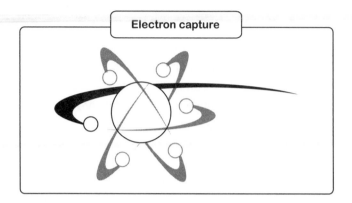

This sets off chain reactions of 'stealing' electrons, which weaken our cellular defences against disease and infection. Obviously, we need to stop the process by 'wiping up' the free radicals before they can cause any damage.

This is where 'antioxidants' come into the picture. Antioxidants mop up the free radicals, preventing damage (and long-term disease), keeping us healthy and seriously delaying the ageing process.

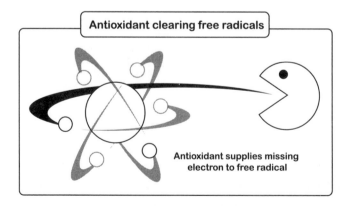

Where do these wondrous things come from? Remember the old expression, 'you are what you eat'? This is where it comes into its own! Antioxidants occur in two main forms:

1. naturally occurring proteins in the body (which we make from essential proteins in our diet)
2. various constituents in our diet which are necessary for the proteins to do their job effectively

The 'various constituents' are essential fatty acids (from eggs, oily fish and certain vegetable oils) and vitamins and minerals (from beef, pork, lamb, poultry, fish, shellfish, fresh fruit, vegetables and dairy products).

You might be able to see a not-very-complicated pattern developing here. If you eat the correct foods to control diabetes, in the correct proportions, you will:

■ improve control of diabetes
■ reduce body fat (naturally) without hunger
■ become much healthier
■ increase your protection against disease and ageing

And all this will cost little or no more than you spend on food at the moment, and take no extra time out of your day. What seemed too good to be true at the start of the book is beginning to make sense, and you can see how easily it can be achieved. It becomes even easier with the suggested recipes later in the book.

VITAMINS AND MINERALS

Vitamins and minerals are essential for health, and we need them in small quantities in our diet. They facilitate certain chemical reactions in our cells, and mop up free radicals, as previously explained. All of the essential vitamins and minerals you need are present in dairy produce, fresh vegetables, tofu and animal foods (beef, pork, lamb, fish, poultry, eggs). And as several of the vitamins are fat-soluble (vitamins A, D, E and K), we need a certain amount of fat in the diet for their effective absorption.

Vitamin A
Typical foods with high concentrations of vitamin A are fish, egg yolk, butter, cheese, carrots, red peppers, spinach, tomatoes and mangetout. Vitamin A is present in most fruits and vegetables, but in varying proportions.

Vitamin B1
Excellent sources of thiamin (vitamin B1) in this diet are pork, fresh fish (especially salmon), certain nuts (cashews, brazils, peanuts, pine nuts) and sesame seeds.

Vitamin B2
Riboflavin (vitamin B2) is present in dairy products (cream and cheese), liver, beef, chicken, eggs, fish, shellfish, mushrooms, avocados and almonds.

Vitamin B3
High concentrations of niacin (vitamin B3) are found in fish (especially salmon and tuna), meat, chicken, liver and eggs.

Vitamin B6

Pyridoxine (vitamin B6) is present in fish (especially tuna), meat (particularly pork), liver, chicken, avocados, nuts (especially walnuts and cashews), tomatoes and tomato purée.

Vitamin B12

Cyanocobalamin (vitamin B12) is the only vitamin not found in foods of plant origin. It is present in highest concentrations in liver, seafood, fish (especially sardines, salmon and tuna), eggs and, in lesser amounts, in milk products and meats.

Folate

The highest concentration of folate occurs in liver, but there are also good amounts in most vegetables (especially green vegetables), meat, poultry, fish, shellfish, eggs and nuts (particularly peanuts and cashews).

Vitamin C

Vitamin C is not present in animal products, apart from liver and kidneys, and has to be obtained from vegetables (especially red and green peppers, mangetout, tomatoes, and broccoli) and fruit (strawberries and citrus fruits).

Vitamin D

This is where oily fish are in a class of their own, providing by far the highest levels of vitamin D compared to any other food group, particularly mackerel, herring, salmon and, to a much lesser degree, tuna. There is a small amount of vitamin D in eggs and butter.

Vitamin E

The requirements for this vitamin are provided in the diet by nuts (almonds, hazelnuts, peanuts), olives, tomato purée, avocados and fish.

Vitamin K

The best dietary source of vitamin K is undoubtedly green vegetables, such as broccoli, cabbage, lettuce, spring onions and spinach.

Minerals

Minerals are natural elements which are necessary for the body's metabolic functions, such as the production of enzymes (selenium) or the manufacture of bones (calcium). These are all present in food. For example:

- Selenium in onions, tomatoes, broccoli, bean sprouts and fish
- Iron in fish, nuts, liver, meat, chicken, sesame seeds and green vegetables
- Manganese in eggs, nuts and green vegetables
- Copper in nuts, mushrooms and green vegetables
- Zinc in eggs, sesame seeds, nuts (especially cashew nuts and almonds), herbs and many vegetables
- Potassium in fish, herbs, garlic, onions, vegetables, mushrooms and citrus fruit
- Calcium in dairy products, fish, green vegetables (especially broccoli and parsley) and herbs
- Sulphur in garlic, onions, fish, eggs, nuts, cabbage and meat

■ ■ ■ ■ ■

You can now appreciate that there are several simple rules you have to follow, and if you do, you will control blood sugars more effectively, reduce body fat, increase body protein and be healthier – all without counting any calories. And for the first time in any diabetic diet you understand what you are doing, and you will be in control!

Chapter 4 Cholesterol – Fact and Fiction

As already explained in Chapter 1, diabetic patients are at a significantly increased risk of various forms of cardiovascular disease, which leads to a greater liability to heart attacks and strokes. A major factor in the development of these conditions is the level of blood cholesterol, which is significantly elevated in diabetic patients. Less well recognised, however, is the fact that these levels can be controlled naturally in a large proportion of patients without the necessity for medication.

Even in patients who need medication to lower cholesterol, improved control of diabetes – by diet – results in a lower requirement for medication. Although the medication used to lower cholesterol (statins) can be very effective, all drugs have potential side effects. As a general rule, the lower the dosage of statins, the lower the complication rate.

What is Cholesterol?

Before discussing the nutritional methods of lowering blood cholesterol, you need to understand what cholesterol is and where it comes from.

The first amazing fact is that most cholesterol in your body is actually made within your body and does not come from diet.

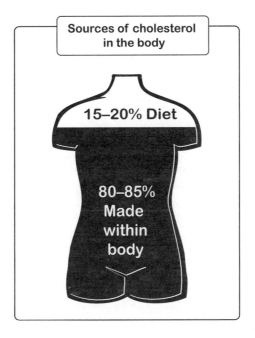

Cholesterol is a fatty substance made by the cells of the body, particularly by the liver, in response to certain stimulants, of which insulin is the most important. So you can see the obvious and instant link with diabetes.

Where is cholesterol found in the body? First, it is important to emphasise that we actually have very little cholesterol in our bodies – only about 150 grams in the whole body and, incredibly, a tiny 7 grams in our blood. Yet these 7 grams in the blood can cause tremendous damage to blood vessels and promote both heart disease and strokes.

Where is the rest of the cholesterol? Most of it is found in the membranes of every cell in your body but other sites include:

- sheaths around nerves
- hormones in the body, particularly the sex hormones
- vitamin D, which regulates calcium and is made from cholesterol
- glands in the skin which keep our skin healthy
- the digestive juices

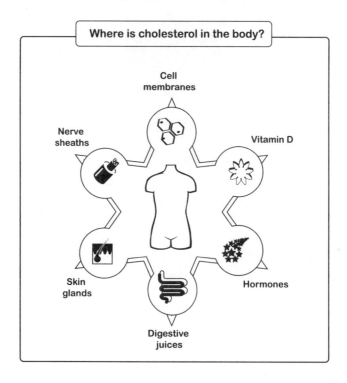

Where is cholesterol in the body?

Cell membranes

Nerve sheaths

Vitamin D

Skin glands

Hormones

Digestive juices

Simply eating less food that contains cholesterol is not the only way to reduce this substance in the blood. However, by reducing your consumption of refined carbohydrates and sugars, you reduce the level of insulin, and, as a direct consequence, the level of cholesterol in your blood is reduced.

'GOOD' AND 'BAD' CHOLESTEROL

There are different types of cholesterol, some of which actually protect your arteries while others cause arterial damage. In simplistic terms, they are really broken into two main categories:

- high density lipoproteins (HDL)
- low density lipoproteins (LDL)

High Density Lipoproteins (HDL) (heart protective)

HDL is a 'good' form of cholesterol which transports fatty deposits away from the arteries and therefore protects against heart disease. These are usually low when insulin levels are elevated and therefore **by lowering insulin levels we increase the amount of protective HDL**, which is obviously very beneficial.

Low Density Lipoproteins (LDL) (heart damage)

LDL is one of the 'bad' forms of cholesterol which can deposit blood fats in the artery walls. **LDL levels are increased when insulin levels are elevated** and therefore, once again, our aim is to lower insulin as much as possible, of which a beneficial side effect is the lowering of LDL levels.

The measurement of total cholesterol in itself is of limited value unless you know how much is 'good' and how much is 'bad'. Obviously, if the cholesterol level is high due to high LDL (bad cholesterol) then our aim would be to lower it as much as possible. However, if a significant proportion of the cholesterol is actually HDL (the protective cholesterol) then our aim is most certainly not to lower the cholesterol. So you can see that it is essential to know the proportion of HDL and LDL in a cholesterol measurement.

TRIGLYCERIDES (HEART DAMAGE)

To confuse the issue even more, cholesterol is not the most important blood fat in the potential development of heart disease. In fact, the blood fats that have this distinction are known as triglycerides. These are produced mainly in your liver in response to insulin. So, once again, by reducing your level of insulin, you reduce the level of triglycerides quite quickly, together with the risk of heart disease.

Cholesterol and Your Diet

Reducing the level of insulin is the single most important factor in lowering the risk of heart disease in diabetic patients. And insulin is reduced by excluding refined carbohydrates from your diet.

Does this mean that you can follow a high-fat diet? Certainly not. The Diabetes Revolution is not a high-fat diet. It is a diet which includes a reasonable proportion of healthy fats, and completely excludes all of the dangerous trans fats present in many processed foods.

This diet is suitable for most diabetic patients. You can lower your serum cholesterol and triglyceride levels by cutting down on refined carbohydrates in your diet and therefore reducing your requirement for insulin. However, some diabetics also have familial hypercholesterolaemia, a form of raised cholesterol in the blood which is predetermined genetically. In other words, they have a higher cholesterol level completely unrelated to diet or lifestyle. In those individuals, it is necessary to lower the level of fats in the diet even more, in addition to following this diet.

Once you start eating a diet low in refined carbohydrates, you can expect to see results quickly. Serum insulin and triglyceride levels will fall within two weeks. HDL is slightly slower and changes may take up to six weeks, and LDL is the slowest of all with the maximum reductions taking three to four months.

In the majority of diabetic patients, the amount of blood fats will be reduced simply by lowering the intake of refined carbohydrates and replacing them with nutritious, healthy foods. For patients who also need to reduce their levels of dietary fat, it is important to realise that cholesterol is only present in foods of animal origin. There is no cholesterol in plant-based foods.

To summarise:

- Cholesterol is a fatty substance in the blood that can cause immense damage to our blood vessels and heart.

- This damage is caused by a relatively tiny amount of cholesterol, only 7 grams of cholesterol in all of the blood vessels in the body.
- Total cholesterol is the sum of all the cholesterol fractions in the blood and is of limited value as a measurement unless we know how much is good cholesterol and how much is bad cholesterol.
- The good cholesterol is HDL and this helps to clean up the arteries.
- The bad cholesterol is LDL and this tends to block the arteries.
- The most dangerous blood fats are triglycerides, and these can be effectively lowered by reducing the refined carbohydrates in our diet.

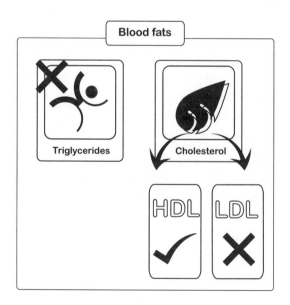

So you can see how essential it is for diabetic patients to reduce their levels of insulin – either as a requirement for injections for a type 1 diabetic or lowering the serum level of insulin in type 2 diabetes – in order to reduce the level of blood fats and therefore lower the risks of heart disease and strokes. And this is all very feasible by nutrition alone in the majority of patients.

Chapter 5 Lowering Blood Sugar Levels

Every diabetic patient knows how important it is to keep their blood sugar level within certain safe limits, but do you know why? Why is a high blood sugar level so dangerous? What are the effects of low blood sugar?

The answer is in two parts: the control of blood sugar in the short term and the effects of poor control in the long term.

Immediate Effects of Poor Blood Sugar Control

HIGH BLOOD SUGAR (HYPERGLYCAEMIA)

In type 1 diabetics, if the blood sugar becomes high this can lead to a very dangerous condition called 'ketoacidosis'. If not treated quickly, it can be fatal and is the commonest cause of death in diabetic patients aged below 20. This is a medical emergency and it is essential for the patient to be admitted to hospital immediately.

In type 2 diabetes the symptoms of high blood sugar are fortunately less dramatic. The usual warning symptoms are:

- thirst
- passing too much urine
- weight loss
- lethargy
- irritability
- blurred vision
- poor concentration
- mood changes

Treatment usually involves adjusting medication or diet, although additional insulin may be required.

LOW BLOOD SUGAR (HYPOGLYCAEMIA)

Low blood sugar (hypoglycaemia) can be caused by a number of different factors. The most common reasons are:

- too little food
- too much exercise
- stress
- high insulin levels, from either
  - too much injected insulin in type 1 diabetes
  or
  - too much insulin produced by the pancreas in type 2 diabetes

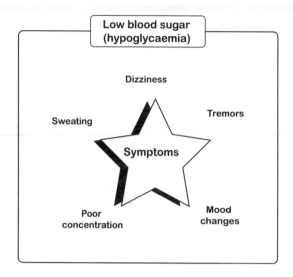

Treatment is effectively achieved by taking glucose tablets and/or a sweet drink (such as Lucozade). Much more important, however, is to identify the cause of the low blood sugar (such as a delayed meal or a particularly strenuous exercise routine) and take action to prevent this happening in the future.

Long-term Effects of Poor Blood Sugar Control

The long-term effects of blood sugar control only relate to high blood sugar. While low blood sugar is essentially only a short-term problem, persistently higher-than-normal blood sugar has very serious long-term consequences.

SUGAR AND PROTEINS

The problem, quite simply, is that when we have too much sugar in our body, the sugar molecules attach themselves to proteins, which form the basic structure of blood vessels, cartilage and skin.

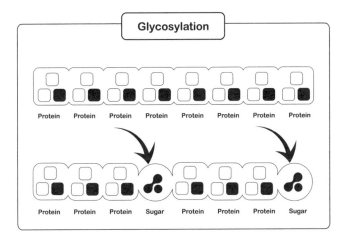

When the sugars attach to these proteins (known as 'glycosylation') this causes hardening of the arteries, reduced elasticity of the skin (causing wrinkling), and stiffening of the joints.

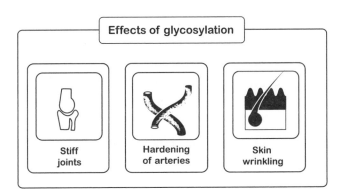

All organs depend on blood vessels for nutrition and oxygen, so damage to blood vessels can lead to significant complications in every organ of the body.

Sugars that attach to proteins are known as Advanced Glycosylation End-products. As you will appreciate, this can be abbreviated to the word 'AGE' – which is very descriptive, as ageing is precisely what these end-products cause. So you can see how important it is to lower blood sugar and prevent this damage to structural proteins in the body.

Glycosylation also causes immense damage within the cells of the body. Although the function of structural proteins is very obvious, forming the structures we can see (bones, cartilage, blood vessels, skin and so on), the proteins within each individual cell are even more important in regulating the millions of chemical processes that occur every second of the day. This means that if the chemical reactions within the cell become affected, the health of every cell in the body is jeopardised, which can lead to premature ageing, sickness and possibly worse.

SUGAR AND RED BLOOD CELLS

Although you may not have heard previously of Advanced Glycosylation End-products, almost all diabetics are aware of the term 'glycosylated haemoglobin' or HbA_{1c}. This is a measurement taken by many diabetics on a regular basis to determine the long-term control of diabetes. It involves measuring the amount of sugar attachment to haemoglobin in the red blood cells of the body. Glycosylated haemoglobin is, quite simply, another of the Advanced Glycosylation

End-products, in other words the attachment of sugar to structural protein in the red blood cells.

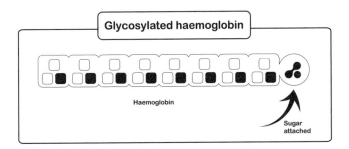

Glycosylated haemoglobin is a reflection of the amount of glycosylation within the whole body. In other words, if diabetes is not well controlled, this process of glycosylation (the disruption of proteins) is occurring throughout the entire body, of which the glycosylated haemoglobin is only one part. So you can now appreciate that glycosylated haemoglobin is much more than just a measure of the control of diabetes: it is an excellent indicator of the disruption of proteins throughout the body by excess sugar.

OTHER EFFECTS OF EXCESS SUGAR

Free Radical Formation

Another particularly dangerous feature of a build-up of excess sugar by glycosylation is that it affects the proteins that protect against free radical formation, the antioxidant proteins in the body (see Chapter 3). Glycosylation of these proteins can result in reduced efficacy of the antioxidants, and if the antioxidant level is low, the level of free radicals in the body is increased. As you have seen earlier, free radical formation is particularly dangerous as it can damage so many cells and accelerate the ageing process.

Raising Bad Cholesterol

The glycosylation process can even affect the formation of the dangerous cholesterol products – the low density lipoproteins – causing LDL to be increased and therefore increasing the risk of heart disease.

■ ■ ■ ■ ■

Probably for the first time, you can now appreciate how desperately important it is to keep blood sugar levels within normal limits. There is no doubt whatsoever that increased levels of blood sugar cause glycosylation of body proteins, weakening the structural proteins and seriously damaging the proteins that control chemical reactions throughout the body. The net effect of this is sickness, premature ageing, detrimental effects on lifestyle and almost certainly a reduction in life expectancy.

All of this can be significantly improved by:

- reducing refined carbohydrates in your diet and therefore lowering the requirement for insulin
- reducing or eliminating all dangerous trans fats from your diet
- taking more exercise

Chapter 6 Type 1 Diabetes: the Programme

In type 1 diabetes, the diet has to be introduced gradually, first with breakfast and lunch, adding dinner about a week later.

Before You Start

You must inform your doctor of proposed changes to your diet and keep them informed of any alterations in medication. All changes must be with your doctor's approval.

Before starting the diet, it is essential to take baseline measurements as follows:

1. Prepare a chart according to the diagram overleaf.
2. Fill in the chart for three days. Take blood glucose measurements before breakfast, lunch, dinner and bedtime. Record the type and amount of insulin injected, the time of each meal and the food consumed.

The chart provides the baseline measurements of your current insulin regime related to your blood glucose.

DATE	TIME	BLOOD GLUCOSE MEASUREMENT	TYPE & AMOUNT OF INSULIN INJECTED	TIME OF MEAL	FOOD CONSUMED

You can now commence the programme!

Week 1

- Continue to fill in the chart recording your blood glucose measurement, insulin and meal details (see above). This will enable you to visualise the effects of reducing refined carbohydrates on your blood glucose and insulin levels. It will also allow you to gauge accurately how much to lower the amount of insulin injected.
- Follow the programme for breakfast and lunch only.
- **Dinner should be your normal high-carbohydrate meal.** This is because your blood sugar levels will reduce quickly on this dietary programme and it is important **to prevent hypoglycaemic episodes during the night**.
- Adjust short-acting insulins (such as Humalog, Novorapid) according to the results of the blood glucose measurements. For example, if you take 10 units of Humalog at 8am and your blood glucose level at 12pm has reduced to 4–5 mmol/l, reduce your Humalog at 8am the next day to 8 units.

This is a gradual process. You are achieving a fine balance between controlling blood glucose within normal limits and preventing hypoglycaemic episodes. That is why it is essential to measure blood glucose at least four times a day and adjust insulin accordingly.

Week 2

- Continue to fill in the chart recording your blood glucose measurement, insulin and meal details (see above).
- By the beginning of the second week, your blood glucose levels at 12pm and 6pm should be reasonably well controlled (5.5–7 mmol/l).
- If these levels are not yet well controlled, prolong the first stage of the programme until this has been achieved.
- **It is absolutely essential that you achieve control of blood glucose at 12pm and 6pm before moving on to the next stage.**
- Assuming that control at 12pm and 6pm has been achieved (with an associated reduction in the amount of insulin injected), you can now move on to the next stage. This is a little more difficult as we have to lower the blood glucose overnight and it is **absolutely essential to prevent hypoglycaemic episodes at night.**
- For this reason, when you add dinner to the dietary regime, **reduce both short-acting and long-acting insulin.** Most patients are prescribed a combination of three short-acting insulins (such as Humalog, Novorapid) with a long-acting insulin (such as Levemir, Lantus). The short-acting insulin injected at 6pm (approximately) will have maximal effects up to between 10pm and midnight. On the other hand, the long-acting insulin, taken at 8–9pm, will have effects until the next evening (24 hours).
- You will have a reasonable estimate of how much to reduce the short-acting insulin by, from your experience during the day.
- The long-acting insulin should be reduced by about 20 per cent initially **but it is important to be aware of the**

possibility of hypoglycaemic episodes at night until the correct dosage is achieved, usually within a few days.

■ In this context, **have precautions available to counteract hypoglycaemia (such as glucose tablets or Lucozade) and inform partners to be aware of the possibility before commencing the second stage of the diet.**

■ Providing your diabetes was reasonably stable at the beginning of the programme, you should be achieving stability at the lower glucose level and lower insulin level within about three weeks.

The Initial Phase Menu Plans

The following menu plans are designed to be guidelines only, and not set in tablets of stone. The only absolute requirements are that you adhere to the 'Principles of the Programme' explained in Chapter 2 (page 32). Of course, if you wish to be certain that you are keeping to the diet, use only the recipes in the book.

All the recipes are explained in detail and simple to prepare, and can be easily adapted to suit every taste. Follow the programme below and control your diabetes!

As already explained on page 65, the Diabetes Revolution is made up of two phases for people with type 1 diabetes. This is because it is essential to prevent hypoglycaemic attacks overnight.

WEEK 1

Our initial aim is to control blood sugars during the day for the first week by appropriately reducing the level of injected insulin before breakfast and lunch.

It is essential that dinner remains a high-carbohydrate meal in the first week of the diet.

By measuring blood sugar immediately before lunch and dinner, you gain the necessary information to control insulin levels before breakfast and lunch respectively: four hours after the injection of short-acting insulin.

WEEK 2

In the second week of the diet (when the high-carbohydrate evening meal is replaced by a low-GI meal), the amount of evening (6pm) short-acting injected insulin (such as Humalog/Novorapid) will initially be reduced by 20 per cent, although this may need to be reduced further depending on the level of morning fasting blood sugar. If morning fasting sugar levels are too low, reduce the level of evening insulin accordingly.

It is essential to prevent hypoglycaemia overnight, which can occur if the insulin level is too high. As you reduce the amount of carbohydrate in your evening meal, the insulin injected must be reduced at the same time.

In addition, long-acting insulin (such as Levemir) will be reduced by about 20 per cent, although further reductions may be necessary depending on the morning fasting sugar levels.

MENU PLAN

Breakfast

Select one from the following:

 Quick-and-easy Muesli (page 106)
Fresh Fruit with Natural Yoghurt (page 106)
Porridge (page 108)
Omelette with various fillings (page 109)
Char-grilled Mushrooms with Scrambled Eggs (page 111)
Eggs Florentine (page 113)
Toasted Cheese (page 115)
Spinach and Cheese Toastie (page 116)
Gruyère and Tomato Toastie (page 117)
Bacon (2 rashers) and eggs (1–2)

Lunch

Month 1

Lunch in the first month of the diet must consist of salad, but you can add protein if you wish. This can include meat (such as ham), egg, chicken, fish (such as smoked salmon), shellfish or cheese.

A selection of delicious salads is described in Chapter 10. However, you can design your own recipes by following the 'Principles of the Programme' in Chapter 2 on page 32. Keep to the rules and the variations are endless.

Month 2

During the second month, you can either maintain a salad regime for lunch or replace it with a more extensive menu. The following are suggestions but the only absolute requirement is that, once again, you keep to the 'Principles of the Programme' on page 32.

 Beef Korma (page 153)

Beefburgers with Herbs (page 155)

Chicken and Ginger (page 165)

Chicken Breast with Chilli Sauce (page 166)

Breast of Chicken with Savoury Filling (page 168)

Citrus Chicken Kebabs (page 170) with baby squash

Turkey and Avocado (page 172)

Salmon Steaks with Leek and Lemon Butter Sauce (page 179)

Salmon with Rocket and Mint Sauce (page 180)

Teriyaki Salmon Kebabs with Cucumber Dip (page 181)

Smoked Salmon with Fennel and Dill (page 182)

Smoked Haddock Soufflé (page 183)

Taramasalata (page 185)

Poached Whiting with Ginger (page 186)

Char-grilled Swordfish with Mustard Dressing (page 188)

Fillets of Dover Sole with Creamy Mushroom Sauce (page 193)

Chilli Tiger Prawns (page 196)

Seared Scallops with Rocket Salad (page 197)

Scallop and Calamari Salad (page 198)

Calamari and Scallops with Flat Mushrooms (page 199)

For Vegetarians

Most of the recipes included on pages 201–219 are suitable for lunch. Additionally, you can have most of the salads on pages 135–147 as a main course. If you like, you can have a side salad with your lunch without disturbing your diabetic control. Many of the non-vegetarian recipes can be adapted by replacing the meat with vegetarian alternatives, such as Quorn.

Dinner

Week 1

You must not eat a low-carbohydrate dinner during Week 1 of the diet. In effect, this means that all of the recipes included on pages 135–219 are excluded during the first week. Dinner recipes in the first week must include higher-GI foods such as:

- bread
- pasta
- rice
- potatoes/parsnips
- cereals/grains

Typical examples of suitable meals are those included in the maintenance phase of the diet (see Chapter 17). These are:

 Penne Rigate with Mixed Veggies (page 229)
Fettucine with Chicken and Basil (page 230)
Pecorino Fettucine with Herbs (page 232)
Tagliatelli Carbonara (page 233)
Wholemeal Spaghetti Napolitana (page 234)
Penne with Char-grilled Vegetables (page 235)
Pappardelle with Two Cheese Sauce (page 236)
Spaghetti Bolognese (page 237)
Lasagne (page 238)
Classic Macaroni Cheese (page 239)

Angel Hair Pasta with Italian Sauce (page 240)

Milanese Risotto (page 241)

Button Mushroom and Basil Risotto (page 242)

Chilli Con Carne (page 243)

Smoked Haddock Kedgeree (page 244)

Chow Mein (page 245)

Week 2

During the second week of the programme, dinner becomes low GI. Therefore, all of the recipes included in the maintenance phase of the diet (pages 227–261) are excluded.

By this stage you will have reduced blood sugars at lunch and dinner, together with appropriate reductions in the amount of short-acting insulin injections. Now you are going to reduce the late afternoon short-acting insulin and, in many cases, the long-acting insulin overnight.

Typical recipes for dinner include all those on pages 135–219. For example:

 Barbecue Thai Lamb (page 148)

Beef Korma (page 153)

Chicken and Ginger (page 165)

Peking Duck (page 176)

Salmon Steaks with Leek and Lemon Butter Sauce (page 179)

Salmon with Rocket and Mint Sauce (page 180)

Smoked Haddock Soufflé (page 183)

Taramasalata (page 185)

Poached Whiting with Ginger (page 186)

Chilli Tiger Prawns (page 196)

Scallop and Calamari Salad (page 198)

Ginger Scallops with Rocket (page 200)

Stir-fried Tofu with Mushrooms (page 201)

Fresh Asparagus with Lemon Butter Sauce (page 202)

Mozzarella Aubergine Slices with Pesto Sauce (page 205)

Spinach with Chilli and Pine Nuts (page 207)

Pepperonata (page 209)

Herb Tomatoes (page 211)

During this phase of the diet, you will be reducing your late-night (pre-dinner) short-acting insulin by about 20 per cent initially, and the long-acting insulin by about 20 per cent. However, it is very likely that these insulins will have to be reduced further as the carbohydrate load is significantly reduced. Every diabetic patient is different and needs to gauge their individual insulin needs.

If you are experiencing significant hunger in late afternoon, this is due to hypoglycaemia and may take some time to resolve over the first few days of the diet. At this time, by far the most effective way to overcome hunger yet maintain control of blood sugar is to have a little smoked salmon with lemon juice, or some cooked chicken (drumsticks, thighs or breast).

Additionally, you can purchase small pots from the deli section in most supermarkets, such as:

- smoked salmon with cream cheese
- chicken with sweetcorn
- tuna mayo

Typical Menu Plan: Type 1 Diabetes, Week 1

	MONDAY	TUESDAY	WEDNESDAY	THURSDAY	FRIDAY	SATURDAY	SUNDAY
Breakfast	Omelette	Spinach and Cheese Toastie	Quick-and-easy Muesli	Emmental Baked Eggs	Porridge	Kippers with Tomatoes	Bacon and eggs
Lunch	Chicken, with Fennel and Tomato Salad	Smoked salmon, with Caper and Olive Salad	Rocket and Olive Salad	Calamari salad	Ham, with Mozzarella and Olive Salad	Prawn mayonnaise, with Green Salad	Rocket and Tofu Salad
Dinner	Penne Rigate with Mixed Veggies	Milanese Risotto	Fettucine with Chicken and Basil	Smoked Haddock Kedgeree	Wholemeal Spaghetti Napolitana	Tagliatelli Carbonara	Chilli Con Carne

Typical Menu Plan: Type 1 Diabetes, Week 2

	MONDAY	TUESDAY	WEDNESDAY	THURSDAY	FRIDAY	SATURDAY	SUNDAY
Breakfast	Omelette	Spinach and Cheese Toastie	Quick-and-easy Muesli	Emmental Baked Eggs	Porridge	Kippers with Tomatoes	Bacon and eggs
Lunch	Mozzarella and Olive Salad	Chicken, with Caper and Olive Salad	Rocket and Olive Salad	Tuna mayonnaise, with Red Lettuce Salad	Ham with cherry tomatoes, and Bocconcini and Parmesan Salad	Prawns, with Watercress, Spinach and Avocado Salad	Warm Beef Salad
Dinner	Salmon with Rocket and Mint Sauce	Ratatouille	Chicken and Ginger	Barbecue Thai Lamb	Smoked Salmon with Fennel and Dill	Seared Scallops with Rocket Salad	Pork Chops with Beetroot Salsa

A little of these foods in late afternoon will resolve hunger, keep sugar levels low and maintain control of diabetes.

Vegetarian diabetics can replace the meat meals with most of the low-GI meals included in the vegetable section (pages 201–219) or can replace the meat in other recipes with vegetarian alternatives, such as Quorn.

Case Histories

Although this is not meant to be a textbook, it is important to provide typical examples of the effect of the diet in controlling blood sugar in both type 1 and type 2 diabetics, and in reducing the requirement for insulin in type 1 diabetes. The experiences of two patients with type 1 diabetes are described here. In Chapter 7, there are case histories for two patients with type 2 diabetes. In all cases, the results are compared over a six-week period.

CASE 1

This 60-year-old male office worker with a 15-year history of known insulin-dependent diabetes had also had raised cholesterol for approximately 10 years. His typical diet, which had been advised by a dietician specialising in diabetes, was as follows:

Breakfast	**2 slices of toast with diabetic jam or marmalade, or fruit (pineapple or mango)**
Lunch	**Sandwich or grilled chicken and salad bowl**
Dinner	**Cold meat salad**

Fish with potatoes or rice
Chipped potatoes once per week

Six weeks later, his typical diet was as follows:

Breakfast   Porridge oats with coffee, or ham and eggs
                  with grapefruit and coffee
Lunch   Salmon salad with soup, or tuna salad with ¼
                  bread roll
Dinner   Chicken salad with 1 glass of wine, or steak
                  with carrots and peas with tea

His main measurements, before and after starting the diet, were as follows:

	FASTING BLOOD GLUCOSE (MMOL/L)	TOTAL CHOLES- TEROL (MMOL/L)	LDL (MMOL/L)	HDL (MMOL/L)	TRIGLYC- ERIDES (MMOL/L)	WEIGHT (KG)
Before	11.5	5.0	2.8	1.3	1.9	90
After	6.5	4.0	1.8	1.9	0.7	87

Over the six-week period, the reduction in his medication was as follows:

	BEFORE	AFTER
Metformin	850 mg twice a day	Unchanged
Novorapid	14 units at 8am, 12pm and 6pm	10 units at 8am, 12pm and 6pm
Levemir	20 units at night	10 units at night

The patient had much more energy after six weeks. He had lost 3 kg in weight and there were significant reductions in his relevant measurements, particularly:

- fasting blood glucose reduced by 43 per cent
- total cholesterol reduced by 20 per cent
- HDL increased by 46 per cent
- LDL reduced by 35 per cent
- triglycerides reduced by 63 per cent

Of much more importance is the fact that his fasting blood glucose was controlled throughout the day on insulin requirements which are approximately 30 per cent lower than previously. The oral medication (Metformin) remained unchanged.

CASE 2

This 20-year-old female university student was diagnosed with insulin-dependent diabetes six years previously. She had gained a considerable amount of weight over these six years, from approximately 55 kg to 77 kg. Her typical diet before commencing the programme was:

Breakfast	**Porridge or Weetabix**
Mid-morning	**Apple or banana with some dried fruit**
Lunch	**2 pieces of bread with salad or baked potato**
Mid-afternoon	**Biscuit with dried fruit**
Dinner	**Salad bowl with bread or rice or fruit**

Six weeks later, her typical diet was as follows:

Breakfast	Scrambled egg, 2 rashers of bacon and
	1 slice of wholemeal bread
Mid-morning	Nothing
Lunch	Chicken salad with lettuce, courgettes and
	broccoli
Mid-afternoon	Nothing
Dinner	Pork salad with lettuce, cucumber, peppers,
	tomatoes and courgettes

Her main measurements, before and after starting the diet, were as follows:

	FASTING BLOOD GLUCOSE (MMOL/L)	TOTAL CHOLES- TEROL (MMOL/L)	LDL (MMOL/L)	HDL (MMOL/L)	TRIGLYC- ERIDES (MMOL/L)	WEIGHT (KG)
Before	12.7	3.9	1.8	1.8	0.6	79
After	8.2	4.4	1.8	2.4	0.47	75

Reduction in medication over the six-week period was as follows:

	BEFORE	AFTER
Levemir	26 units at 10pm	16 units at 10pm
Novorapid	12–15 units at 8am, 12pm and 6pm	4 units at 8am and 12pm, and 6 units at 6pm

The improvements in control of her diabetes were objectively proved by the following:

- fasting blood glucose reduced by 35 per cent
- HDL increased by 33 per cent
- LDL unchanged
- triglycerides reduced by 22 per cent
- reduction in requirement of Novorapid by 50 per cent and Levemir by 35 per cent

Although her total cholesterol levels actually increased by 13 per cent, this is entirely a result of the protective HDL increasing by 33 per cent while the LDL level remained unchanged. This is an excellent example of the fallacy of depending entirely on recording total cholesterol rather than the breakdown into good and bad cholesterol.

Chapter 7 Type 2 Diabetes: the Programme

This diet is particularly suitable for type 2 diabetes (not requiring insulin) as there is no danger of hypoglycaemia associated with excess insulin injection. On the contrary, the level of insulin produced by your body will decrease on this diet, reducing the risks of obesity, heart disease and strokes linked with elevated insulin levels.

Before You Start

You must inform your doctor of proposed changes to your diet and keep them informed of any alterations in medication. All changes must be with your doctor's approval.

Type 2 diabetics not taking insulin can start the full diet immediately (overleaf), rather than in a staged process as for type 1 diabetics, because there is a low risk of hypoglycaemia.

Type 2 diabetics requiring insulin must adhere to a staged process. Before starting the diet, it is essential to take baseline measurements as follows:

1. Prepare a chart according to the diagram on page 66.
2. Fill in the chart for three days. Take blood glucose measurements before breakfast, lunch, dinner and bedtime. Record the time of each meal and the food consumed, and details of any medication taken.

The chart provides the baseline measurements of your current insulin regime related to your blood glucose.
You can now commence the programme!

Week 1

- Continue to fill in the chart recording your blood glucose measurement, insulin and meal details (see above). This will enable you to visualise the effects of reducing refined carbohydrates on your blood glucose and insulin levels. It will also allow you to gauge accurately how much to lower the amount of insulin injected.
- Follow the programme for breakfast and lunch only.
- **Dinner should be your normal high-carbohydrate meal.** This is because your blood sugar levels will reduce quickly on this dietary programme and it is important **to prevent hypoglycaemic episodes during the night**.
- Adjust short-acting insulins (such as Humalog, Novorapid) according to the results of the blood glucose measurements. For example, if you take 10 units of Humalog at 8am and your blood glucose level at 12pm has reduced to 4–5 mmol/l, reduce your Humalog at 8am the next day to 8 units.

This is a gradual process. You are achieving a fine balance between controlling blood glucose within normal limits and preventing hypoglycaemic episodes. That is why it is essential to measure blood glucose at least four times a day and adjust insulin accordingly.

Week 2

- Continue to fill in the chart recording your blood glucose measurement, medication and meal details (see above).
- By the beginning of the second week, your blood glucose levels at 12pm and 6pm should be reasonably well controlled (5.5–7 mmol/l).
- If these levels are not yet well controlled, prolong the first stage of the programme until this has been achieved (see Chapter 6).
- **It is absolutely essential that you achieve control of blood glucose at 12pm and 6pm before moving on to the next stage.**
- Assuming that control at 12pm and 6pm has been achieved (with an associated reduction in the amount of insulin injected), you can now move on to the next stage. This is a little more difficult as we have to lower the blood glucose overnight and it is **absolutely essential to prevent hypoglycaemic episodes at night**.
- For this reason, when you add dinner to the dietary regime, **reduce both short-acting and long-acting insulin**. The requirements for insulin vary between patients with type 2 diabetes, depending on diabetic control, so it is only possible to discuss the subject in general principles rather than absolute specifics. Patients may be prescribed a

combination of up to three short-acting insulins (such as Humalog, Novorapid) with a long-acting insulin (such as Levemir, Lantus). The short-acting insulin injected at 6pm (approximately) will have maximal effects up to between 10pm and midnight. On the other hand, the long-acting insulin, taken at 8–9pm, will have effects until the next evening (24 hours).

- You will have a reasonable estimate of how much to reduce the short-acting insulin by, from your experience during the day.
- The long-acting insulin should be reduced by about 20 per cent initially **but it is important to be aware of the possibility of hypoglycaemic episodes at night until the correct dosage is achieved, usually within a few days.**
- In this context, **have precautions available to counteract hypoglycaemia (such as glucose tablets or Lucozade) and inform partners to be aware of the possibility before commencing the second stage of the diet.**
- Providing your diabetes was reasonably stable at the beginning of the programme, you should be achieving stability at the lower glucose level and lower insulin level within about three weeks.

The Initial Phase Menu Plans

The following menu plans are designed to be guidelines only, not set in tablets of stone. The only absolute requirements are that you adhere to the 'Principles of the Programme' explained in Chapter 2 (page 32). Of course, if you wish to be certain that you are keeping to the diet, use only the recipes in the book.

All the recipes are explained in detail and simple to prepare, and can be easily adapted to suit every taste. Follow the programme below and control your diabetes!

The dietary programme for type 2 diabetics depends upon whether insulin injection is required or not:

Type 2 diabetics requiring insulin must follow the programme for type 1 diabetics (pages 65–82), with Week 1 of the diet including a high-GI dinner, and proceeding to reduce the evening meal to low GI in Week 2 only.

Type 2 diabetics not requiring insulin (controlled by oral medication alone) can start the diet in full immediately, rather than in a staged process as for type 1 diabetes, because there is a low risk of hypoglycaemia.

Diabetic patients must be aware, however, that insulin levels will lower significantly on this diet, so the need for oral medication will probably be reduced with the improved control of sugar levels. They need to continue to measure their blood sugars on a regular basis and reduce medication accordingly, with their doctor's full knowledge and agreement.

MENU PLAN FOR TYPE 2 DIABETICS NOT REQUIRING INSULIN

The menu plan for type 2 diabetes (not requiring insulin) is exactly the same as for Week 2 of type 1 diabetes (page 70). In other words, there is no need to include high-GI evening meals in the first week as there is a very low risk of hypoglycaemia in type 2 diabetes.

Typical Menu Plan: Type 2 Diabetes

	MONDAY	TUESDAY	WEDNESDAY	THURSDAY	FRIDAY	SATURDAY	SUNDAY
Breakfast	Omelette	Spinach and Cheese Toastie	Quick-and-easy Muesli	Emmental Baked Eggs	Porridge	Kippers with Tomatoes	Bacon and eggs
Lunch	Chicken, with Fennel and Tomato Salad	Smoked salmon, with Caper and Olive Salad	Rocket and Olive Salad	Calamari salad	Ham, with Mozzarella and Olive Salad	Prawn mayonnaise, with Green Salad	Rocket and Tofu Salad
Dinner	Salmon with Rocket and Mint Sauce	Ratatouille	Chicken and Ginger	Barbecue Thai Lamb	Smoked Salmon with Fennel and Dill	Seared Scallops with Rocket Salad	Pork Chops with Beetroot Salsa

Therefore you can include all the breakfast options in Chapter 8 and any of the recipes from the soups, fish, shellfish, meat, poultry, vegetable and salad sections. The only recipes you need to exclude at this stage are those in the maintenance phase (Chapter 17) which are high GI.

If you are experiencing significant hunger in late afternoon, this is due to hypoglycaemia and may take some time to resolve over the first few days of the diet. At this time, by far the most effective way to overcome hunger yet maintain control of blood sugar is to have a little smoked salmon with lemon juice, or some cooked chicken (drumsticks, thighs or breast).

Additionally, you can purchase small pots from the deli section in most supermarkets such as:

- smoked salmon with cream cheese
- chicken with sweetcorn
- tuna mayo

A little of these foods in late afternoon will resolve hunger, keep sugar levels low and maintain control of diabetes.

Case Histories

We have selected two case histories to give you a brief idea of the effects of the Diabetes Revolution on people with type 2 diabetes:

- a type 2 diabetic patient on medication alone
- a type 2 diabetic patient requiring insulin in addition to medication because of poor diabetic control

CASE 1

This 39-year-old female had type 2 diabetes for 12 years, requiring insulin for two years. Her typical diet before starting the programme was as follows:

Breakfast	All Bran or Shreddies with sugar substitute, or porridge
Mid-morning	Cheese and biscuits or bread and Marmite with some fruit (banana, orange or apple)
Lunch	Soup or a sandwich
Mid-afternoon	Fruit or biscuits
Dinner	Pasta with salad, or meat with 2 vegetables, followed by fruit and yoghurt

Six weeks later, her typical diet was as follows:

Breakfast	Porridge, 1 slice of toast and marmalade and tea
Mid-morning	Nothing
Lunch	Soup, 2 pieces of fresh fruit
Mid-afternoon	Nothing
Dinner	Steak with mixed vegetables, yoghurt and blueberries

Her main measurements, before and after starting the diet, were as follows:

	FASTING BLOOD GLUCOSE (MMOL/L)	TOTAL CHOLES-TEROL (MMOL/L)	LDL (MMOL/L)	HDL (MMOL/L)	TRIGLYC-ERIDES (MMOL/L)	WEIGHT (KG)
Before	9.8	4.6	2.1	1.5	2.1	100
After	7.7	3.9	1.6	1.7	1.3	96

Reduction in medication over the six-week period was as follows:

	BEFORE	AFTER
Levemir	40 units at 10pm	30 units at 10pm
Novorapid	12 units at 8am, 14 units at 12pm, 20 units at 6pm	9 units at 8am, 10 units at 12pm, 16 units at 6pm

You can see that the results of diabetic control improved significantly:

- fasting blood glucose reduced by 21 per cent
- total cholesterol reduced by 15 per cent
- LDL reduced by 24 per cent
- HDL increased by 13 per cent
- triglycerides reduced by 38 per cent

And these results were achieved by diet alone, with an associated reduction of Novorapid and Levemir by approximately 25 per cent.

CASE 2

This 48-year-old woman had been diagnosed with type 2 diabetes three years previously. Her diabetes was poorly controlled through diet and 850 mg Metformin three times per day.

Before starting the programme, her typical diet was as follows:

Breakfast	**Porridge (plus 3 teaspoons of sugar) or**
	2 slices of buttered toast
Mid-morning	**Nothing**
Lunch	**Sandwich (2 slices of bread)**
Mid-afternoon	**Tea with chocolate biscuit**
Dinner	**Pasta with meat/fish/chicken plus**
	vegetables (including potatoes)
Before bed	**Chocolate or fruit**

Six weeks later, her typical diet was as follows:

Breakfast	**Omelette**
Mid-morning	**Nothing**
Lunch	**Chicken or tuna salad with dressing**
Mid-afternoon	**Nothing**
Dinner	**Lean steak/fish/chicken plus vegetables**
	1 piece fruit

Her main measurements, before and after starting the diet, were as follows:

	FASTING BLOOD GLUCOSE (MMOL/L)	TOTAL CHOLES- TEROL (MMOL/L)	LDL (MMOL/L)	HDL (MMOL/L)	TRIGLYC- ERIDES (MMOL/L)	WEIGHT (KG)
Before	9.7	4.1	2.5	1.0	1.4	103
After	6.2	2.0	1.9	1.0	0.9	95.5

The main contributing factor to type 2 diabetes is insulin resistance (see page 2); therefore the fasting insulin level is fundamental to managing the disease. In this patient, fasting insulin levels reduced from 33.2 mIU/l to 13.7 mIU/l in only six weeks, a reduction of 58 per cent. As insulin is the major factor controlling the deposition of fat in the body, lowering insulin undoubtedly contributed to the reduction of weight by 7.5 kg in six weeks. There was no specific reduction of calories during this phase, merely the elimination of refined carbohydrates from the diet. In addition, it can be seen that:

- fasting blood glucose reduced by 36 per cent
- total cholesterol reduced by 48 per cent
- HDL remained static
- LDL reduced by 24 per cent
- triglycerides reduced by 35 per cent

Chapter 8 Breakfast

Breakfast Drinks

Although the combination of various fruit and vegetable juices can be delicious, you can also enjoy pure juices of single fruits, either undiluted or with added spring water. Keep the carb count to less than 60 grams per day and the way you enjoy your (healthy) carbs is up to you!

Raspberry and grapefruit (FOR 2)

150 grams raspberries
1 small grapefruit, segmented

■   Juice the raspberries and grapefruit segments and serve immediately.

Carbohydrate content per serving: 9 grams

Melon and blueberries

½ honeydew melon, peeled and segmented
100 grams blueberries, washed

■   Juice the melon and blueberries and serve immediately.

Carbohydrate content per serving: 11 grams

Melon and lemon

½ honeydew melon, peeled, chopped and juiced
Juice of a freshly squeezed lemon
75 ml cold spring water

■   Stir ingredients together. Serve immediately.

Carbohydrate content per serving: 8 grams

Melon and mint FOR 2

1 medium, ripe Galia melon, peeled, deseeded and chopped
3 tbsp freshly squeezed lemon juice
1 tbsp fresh mint leaves
Sprigs of fresh mint, to garnish

■   Purée ingredients, garnish with mint and serve.

Carbohydrate content per serving: 14 grams

Watercress and carrot   (FOR 2)

100 grams watercress
2 large carrots, peeled, topped and tailed and chopped
1 lemon, quartered

- Juice the ingredients and serve immediately.

Carbohydrate content per serving: 8 grams

Carrot and apple   (FOR 2)

1 large carrot, peeled and chopped
1 medium apple, peeled, cored and chopped
1 tsp orange zest

- Juice the carrot, apple and orange zest.
- Serve immediately.

Carbohydrate content per serving: 8 grams

Strawberry and pear   (FOR 2)

100 grams strawberries
1 medium pear, cored, peeled and chopped

- Juice the strawberries and pear segments.
- Serve immediately.

Carbohydrate content per serving: 11 grams

Strawberry and blackberry (FOR 2)

100 grams strawberries, washed and hulled
100 grams blackberries, washed

■   Juice the berries and serve immediately.

Carbohydrate content per serving: 9 grams

Berry zest (FOR 2)

100 grams each blueberries and strawberries
1 tbsp freshly squeezed lime juice
100 ml water

■   Blend together the blueberries, strawberries and lime
juice. Dilute to taste.

Carbohydrate content per serving: 10 grams

Avocado, tomato and basil (FOR 2)

1 small Hass avocado, stone removed, peeled and
chopped
3 medium plum tomatoes on the vine, chopped
6–8 large basil leaves, washed and chopped finely

■   Blend the ingredients and serve immediately.

Carbohydrate content per serving: 4 grams

Peach and orange   (FOR 2)

1 medium peach, stone removed
1 medium orange, peeled, segmented and pips removed

- Juice the peach and orange segments.
- Strain and serve immediately.

Carbohydrate content per serving: 9 grams

Kiwi and orange   (FOR 2)

2 kiwi fruit, peeled and chopped
1 orange, peeled, segmented and pips removed
1 tsp orange zest
6 mint leaves
Sprig of mint, to garnish

- Juice the ingredients.
- Stir and serve immediately, garnished with a sprig of mint.

Carbohydrate content per serving: 12 grams

Citrus stinger

1 medium grapefruit, peeled
2 medium oranges, peeled, segmented and pips removed
1 tbsp freshly squeezed lime juice
50 ml water (optional)

- Juice the fruit and blend together
- Dilute with water, to taste, if desired.

Carbohydrate content per serving: 13 grams

Citrus carrot

2 large Seville oranges, peeled, segmented and pips
    removed
2 tbsp freshly squeezed lemon juice
2 large carrots, topped and tailed, peeled and chopped
50 ml water (optional)

- Blend the carrots and oranges with the lemon juice.
- Dilute with water, to taste.

Carbohydrate content per serving: 10 grams

Citrus and ginger   (FOR 2)

1 medium orange, peeled, segmented and pips removed
3 slices of fresh root ginger, peeled and finely chopped
1 tbsp freshly squeezed lime juice
15 grapes
75 ml water
Sprig of mint, to garnish

- Blend the orange segments, ginger, lime juice and grapes.
- Stir in the cold spring water.
- Serve immediately, garnished with a sprig of mint.

Carbohydrate content per serving: 10 grams

Cucumber and mint surprise   (FOR 2)

1 medium cucumber, peeled, deseeded and chopped
2 tbsp freshly chopped mint leaves
200 ml crème fraîche
1 tbsp freshly squeezed lemon juice
Ice cubes
Mint leaves, to garnish

- Blend the cucumber, chopped mint, crème fraîche and lemon juice until smooth.
- Serve immediately with ice cubes and garnish with mint leaves.

Carbohydrate content per serving: 10 grams

SMOOTHIES

Milk (whether full-fat, semi-skimmed or skimmed) contains approximately 5 grams of carbohydrate per 100 ml. Natural yoghurt contains about 6 grams per 100 ml. By restricting the amount of yoghurt or milk, you can easily include smoothies in your low-GI diet.

Mint and cucumber smoothie   (FOR 2)

1 tbsp chopped mint leaves
1 medium English cucumber, peeled, deseeded and
     chopped
200 ml natural yoghurt

- Blend together the ingredients and serve immediately.

Carbohydrate content per serving: 12 grams

Mango and strawberry smoothie   (FOR 2)

1 ripe mango
100 grams ripe strawberries
125 ml cold full-fat milk

- Juice the mango.
- Blend together the mango juice, strawberries and
  milk.

Carbohydrate content per serving: 14 grams

Raspberry and orange smoothie   (FOR 2)

100 grams raspberries
100 ml natural yoghurt
100 ml freshly squeezed orange juice

- Blend together the raspberries and yoghurt.
- Add the orange juice and blend until smooth.

Carbohydrate content per serving: 9 grams

Mango and lemon smoothie   (FOR 2)

150 ml milk, chilled
1 medium fresh mango, peeled, stone removed and
    chopped
2 tbsp freshly squeezed lemon juice
2 tsp runny honey
Fresh mint leaves, to garnish

- Blend together the milk, mango, lemon juice and
  honey until smooth.
- Serve immediately, garnished with fresh mint leaves.

Carbohydrate content per serving: 25 grams

Berry surprise (FOR 2)

100 grams blackberries
100 grams blueberries
100 ml natural yoghurt, chilled
Crushed ice

- Blend together the blackberries, blueberries, yoghurt and ice.
- Serve immediately.

Carbohydrate content per serving: 16 grams

Citrus smoothie (FOR 2)

3 tbsp freshly squeezed lemon juice
2 tbsp freshly squeezed lime juice
2 tsp caster sugar
150 ml natural yoghurt, chilled

- Blend together the lemon juice, lime juice, caster sugar and yoghurt.
- Serve immediately.

Carbohydrate content per serving: 11 grams

Strawberry and whey smoothie   (FOR 2)

150 grams strawberries (or raspberries)
50 grams whey protein powder
100 ml water

- Blend together the strawberries, whey protein and water.
- Serve immediately.

Carbohydrate content per serving: 12 grams

Carb Content of Fruits

	CARB GRAMS
Apple	10
Apricot	7
Blackberries (100 g)	12
Blueberries (100 g)	13
Cherries (100 g)	12
Gooseberries (100 g)	13
Grapefruit (100 g)	10
Grapes (100 g)	
Black grapes	15
Green grapes	12
Kiwi fruit	7
Lemon	3
Lime	1
Mandarin	4
Melon (100 g)	
Honeydew	6
Rock	5
Watermelon	5
Nectarine	7
Orange	10
Passion fruit	3
Peach	8
Pear	16
Pineapple (100 g)	8
Plum	8
Raspberries (100 g)	5
Rhubarb (100 g)	1
Strawberries (100 g)	6
Tangerine	7

Cold Breakfasts

Quick-and-easy muesli   (FOR 2)

60 grams rolled oats
100 ml apple juice
1 medium red apple, peeled, cored and grated
200 ml chilled natural yoghurt
1 tsp ground cinnamon

- Mix together the rolled oats and apple juice in a medium bowl and soak for 2–3 hours in the fridge.
- Stir in the grated apple.
- Stir in the yoghurt, sprinkle with cinnamon and serve immediately.

Carbohydrate content per serving: 37 grams

Fresh fruit with natural yoghurt   (FOR 2)

1 medium red apple, peeled, cored and chopped
1 medium orange, peeled, deseeded and chopped
100 grams fresh strawberries, washed and hulled
100 ml natural yoghurt

- Mix together the chopped apple, orange and strawberries in a medium bowl.
- Transfer to breakfast bowls, pour over the yoghurt and serve immediately.

Carbohydrate content per serving: 19 grams

Breakfast platter

A delicious breakfast platter can be simple or diverse, according to taste. Almost all of the foods can be purchased ready to eat (except boiled eggs, which will only take a few minutes) so this has to be the ultimate fast breakfast. And as all of the foods are low GI and low in sugar (apart from fruit), they are perfectly suited to improving your diabetic control. Typical examples of appropriate foods include:

- fresh deli ham, turkey, chicken or beef
- continental salamis and sausages (maximum of 50 grams)
- natural cheeses (the only exceptions are some processed cheeses)
- smoked fish: mackerel, haddock, salmon or kippers
- hard-boiled eggs
- chicken: legs, thighs or breast
- nuts (restricted to 50 grams per day): especially almonds, walnuts, brazil nuts and hazelnuts – but excluding peanuts, cashew and pistachio nuts
- 1 piece of fruit (or a bowl of berries with natural yoghurt) but excluding bananas, mangos and pineapples

Hot breakfasts

Porridge   (FOR 2)

400 ml water, boiled
3 tbsp oatmeal
2 tsp granulated sugar (optional)
8 tbsp full-cream milk

- Pour the water into a medium saucepan, bring to the boil and stir in the oatmeal.
- Simmer gently for 20–25 minutes.
- Mix in the sugar, if desired, and milk and serve immediately.

Carbohydrate content per serving: 25 grams (20 grams without added sugar)

Omelette

4 large, fresh free-range eggs
2 tbsp full-cream milk
Pinch of rock salt
Freshly ground black pepper
30 grams unsalted butter

- Beat the eggs in a medium mixing bowl, add the milk and season to taste.
- Heat the butter in a medium omelette pan, add the egg mixture and allow to cook on high for about a minute, then gently lift the edges of the omelette with a spatula, allowing the egg to cook more rapidly.
- When the egg just begins to set, but is still creamy, fold the sides of the omelette to the centre, and serve immediately.

Here are a few suggested fillings:

- Parma ham (diced), diced plum tomato and chives
- chopped fresh basil and coriander
- freshly grated Gruyère and chives, garnished with freshly grated Parmesan
- asparagus and basil
- finely chopped cooked chicken breast with tarragon
- diced smoked salmon with dill
- diced and deseeded red and yellow peppers
- sliced mushrooms (pre-cooked) with chopped tomato and chopped fresh oregano

Carbohydrate content per serving: 1–4 grams (depending on filling)

Perfect scrambled eggs (FOR 2)

2 eggs
3 tbsp cream
Freshly ground black pepper
25 grams butter

- Whisk together the eggs and cream in a medium mixing bowl and season to taste.
- Melt the butter in a medium frying pan and add the egg mixture.
- As the egg begins to set around the edges, stir continuously then serve immediately.

All of the fillings appropriate for omelettes (page 109) can also be added to scrambled eggs for improved taste and nutrition.

Carbohydrate content per serving: 1–4 grams (depending on filling)

Char-grilled mushrooms with scrambled eggs

1 tbsp unsalted butter
1 tbsp Dijon mustard
2 large Portobello mushrooms
2 large free-range eggs
1 tbsp freshly chopped basil
1 tbsp freshly chopped chives
Freshly ground black pepper

- Melt the butter in a small saucepan and mix in the Dijon mustard.
- Spread the mixture over the mushrooms and grill under a hot grill (no closer than 8–10 cm from the grill) for about 5 minutes.

At the same time:

- Prepare the scrambled eggs (opposite).
- Stir the basil into the scrambled eggs.
- Place the mushrooms in the centre of each plate and top with scrambled eggs.
- Garnish with chopped chives and season to taste.

Carbohydrate content per serving: 3 grams

Emmental baked eggs (FOR 2)

4 medium free-range eggs
50 grams butter
2 slices honey mustard ham, finely chopped
2 tbsp finely chopped fresh basil
2 tbsp Emmental cheese, freshly grated

- Preheat the oven to 180°C (gas mark 4).
- Whisk the eggs in a medium mixing bowl.
- Mix together the honey mustard ham and basil.
- Butter 4 ramekins and spoon the ham and basil mixture evenly between them.
- Fill the ramekins with the egg mixture and sprinkle over the cheese.
- Place the ramekins in a roasting tin half full of water and cook in the centre of the oven for 25–30 minutes.
- Remove the ramekins from the oven and serve immediately.

Carbohydrate content per serving: 2 grams

Eggs Florentine

75 grams unsalted butter
500 grams fresh spinach leaves, rinsed, drained and stalks
    removed
2 tbsp chopped fresh basil leaves
4 large, fresh free-range eggs
2 tbsp Parmesan cheese, grated
Freshly ground black pepper

- Preheat the oven to 180°C (gas mark 4).
- Melt the butter in a large saucepan, then gently sauté the spinach and basil over a low heat for 1–2 minutes until just softened (not too long, or it will disappear!)
- Transfer the spinach mixture to a shallow, oven-safe dish and smooth evenly over the base.
- Form 4 hollow shapes in the spinach and break an egg into the centre of each hollow.
- Sprinkle ½ tbsp of Parmesan cheese over each egg, season to taste and cook in the centre of the oven for 12–15 minutes.
- Serve immediately.

Carbohydrate content per serving: 6 grams

Poached eggs   (FOR 2)

2 large free-range eggs

You can poach eggs either by the traditional method or, if time is of the essence in the morning, more rapidly by microwave.

By microwave
Break each egg individually into the plastic cups specially designed for microwave poaching of eggs. Pierce the top of the yolks 4–5 times with a sharp knife, add a teaspoon of cold water and close the sealed top of the cup. Cook on medium (careful, on 'high' it will explode!) for about 1–2 minutes (depending on the power of the microwave), then allow to stand for another minute before serving.

Traditional method
Heat the water to boiling point in a shallow pan then reduce the heat to a gentle simmer. Break each egg individually into a cup, and slide the eggs gently into the boiling water. Cook for approximately 3–4 minutes, removing the eggs from the water with a perforated spoon when the yolk is evenly coated with a white film, and the white has cooked. Serve on a slice of buttered wholemeal toast.

Carbohydrate content per serving: negligible (without toast);
17 grams (with toast)

Toasted cheese   (FOR 2)

2 slices of wholemeal bread
1 large plum tomato, sliced
50 grams freshly grated cheese (try Wensleydale, Edam,
        Jarlsberg, Cheddar or Halloumi)
1 tsp Worcester sauce
Freshly ground black pepper

- Lightly toast one side of the wholemeal bread.
- Arrange the slices of tomato on the other side,
  sprinkle over the cheese and drizzle over a few drops
  of Worcester sauce.
- Season with freshly ground black pepper, and lightly
  grill until the cheese melts.

Carbohydrate content per serving: 18 grams

Spinach and cheese toastie (FOR 2)

25 grams butter
50 grams baby spinach leaves
2 slices wholemeal bread
4 slices Emmental cheese
Freshly ground black pepper

- Melt the butter in a medium saucepan and sauté the spinach until it just begins to soften.

At the same time:

- Toast the bread.
- Top the bread with the sautéed spinach.
- Place the Emmental slices on top and grill under a medium heat until the cheese begins to melt.
- Season to taste and serve immediately.

Carbohydrate content per serving: 18 grams

Gruyère and tomato toastie (FOR 2)

2 slices of wholemeal bread, lightly toasted
4 plum tomatoes on the vine, sliced
50 grams grated Gruyère cheese
½ Hass avocado, peeled, stone removed and finely sliced
Freshly ground black pepper

- Place the tomato slices on the toasted bread, top with grated cheese and grill under a medium grill (8–10 cm from the grill) for 2–3 minutes.
- Serve immediately with sliced avocado and black pepper.

Carbohydrate content per serving: 24 grams

Kippers with tomatoes (FOR 2)

3 tbsp extra-virgin olive oil
2 medium kippers
4 medium plum tomatoes, sliced
Freshly ground black pepper

- Heat the olive oil in a medium frying pan and add the kippers.
- Cook the kippers for 4–5 minutes, turning once, then add the tomatoes and cook for a further minute.
- Season to taste and serve immediately.

Carbohydrate content per serving: 5 grams

Crêpes (FOR 2)

Each crêpe contains only 5–6 grams of carbohydrate (or about one-third of the amount in a single slice of bread) so they are perfect for a low-GI diet. This recipe can be made by hand, or using a blender. The variety of potential toppings is almost infinite: see the recipe opposite for a suggestion.

50 grams plain flour
Pinch of salt
1 large free-range egg, beaten
150 ml full-cream milk
1 tbsp melted butter

- Sieve the flour and salt into a medium bowl.
- Add half the beaten egg mixture, whisking constantly.
- Gradually blend in the milk, drawing the mixture to the centre of the bowl until you achieve an even consistency.
- Allow to stand for at least half an hour before making the crêpes.
- Just before cooking, stir the melted butter into the mixture.

Crêpes can be cooked by either the traditional method or using a commercial crêpe-maker. Crêpe-makers are not expensive, and effectively allow you to make crêpes quickly and include them regularly in your low-carb diet.

Traditional method
- Add 1 level tbsp of butter to a small non-stick frying pan, melt the butter over a medium heat and evenly coat the pan.

- Add 2 tbsp of the mixture to the pan then tip the pan to evenly coat the base.
- Cook for about 20–30 seconds and remove with a pallete knife.

Crêpe-maker

- Pour the mixture into a wide shallow dish.
- Turn on the crêpe-maker. When hot, dip the crêpe-maker horizontally on to the mixture to lightly coat and allow the crêpe to cook. When the edge of the crêpe is lightly browned, remove with a palette knife and repeat the process.

Egg and pancetta crêpe (FOR 2)

6 crêpes (see opposite)
2 medium free-range eggs
4 slices of pancetta
Freshly ground black pepper
1 tbsp chopped fresh flat-leaf parsley

- Prepare the crêpes and scramble or poach the eggs.

At the same time:

- Grill the pancetta.
- Fold the crêpes into triangles, place 3 on each plate and top with pancetta and eggs.
- Season to taste and garnish with parsley.

Carbohydrate content per serving: 21 grams

Caramelised apples with pineapple and mint   (FOR 2)

2 large Royal Gala apples (or similar, to taste)
25 grams unsalted butter
Pinch of cinnamon
100 grams fresh pineapple, chopped
1 tbsp chopped fresh mint leaves

- Peel and core the apples then slice finely, place on a grill-tray and dot with butter.
- Cook under a medium grill (no closer than 8–10 cm to the heat) for 2–3 minutes, turning once.
- Sprinkle over a little cinnamon, spoon the chopped pineapple on to the apple and garnish with fresh mint. Serve immediately.

Carbohydrate content per serving: 18 grams

Chapter 9 Soups

Soups are a great source of nutrition. Being low GI, they are an excellent way to bring diabetes under control.

Carrot and coriander soup (FOR 2)

1 tbsp extra-virgin olive oil
3 shallots, peeled and chopped
4 large carrots, scraped and chopped
400 ml Swiss bouillon vegetable stock
Freshly ground black pepper
2 tbsp chopped fresh coriander

- Heat the olive oil in a medium saucepan and sauté the shallots for about 3–4 minutes.
- Add the carrots and stock, season with black pepper, bring to the boil and simmer for about 30 minutes.
- Purée the mixture in a blender.
- Return the soup to the saucepan, stir in the coriander and heat gently. Serve immediately.

Carbohydrate content per serving: 12 grams

Tomato and red pepper soup   (FOR 2)

1 tbsp extra-virgin olive oil
4 shallots, peeled and finely chopped
1 large garlic clove, peeled and finely chopped
2 medium red peppers, deseeded and diced
200 grams large vine-ripened tomatoes, blanched, skins
    removed and chopped
400 ml Swiss bouillon vegetable stock
2 slices of fresh root ginger, peeled and chopped
1 tbsp chopped fresh basil
1 tbsp chopped fresh coriander
Freshly ground black pepper
1 tbsp crème fraîche

- Heat the olive oil in a large saucepan.
- Sauté the shallots, garlic and peppers for about
  3–4 minutes.
- Add the tomatoes, stock and ginger, cover and gently
  simmer for approximately 25–30 minutes.
- Purée in a blender until smooth. Return the soup to
  the pan, add the basil and coriander and heat through
  gently.
- Season to taste with freshly ground black pepper.
- Stir in the crème fraîche and serve immediately.

Carbohydrate content per serving: 22 grams

Tomato and basil soup (FOR 2)

A simple method of peeling tomatoes is to put a shallow cross in each tomato at its base. Place the tomatoes in a bowl of boiling water for 30 seconds, then drain off the water. Immerse the tomatoes in cold water for a few seconds and the skins should peel easily. Ripe tomatoes are much easier to peel.

2 tbsp extra-virgin olive oil
350 grams plum tomatoes, peeled and chopped
1 garlic clove, peeled and finely chopped
3 spring onions, finely chopped
2 tbsp chopped fresh basil
1 bay leaf
350 ml chicken or vegetable stock
1 tbsp tomato purée
Freshly ground black pepper
2 tsp cornflour
Pinch of rock salt
100 ml single cream
2 tsp chopped fresh basil, to garnish

- Heat the olive oil in a large saucepan and then add the tomatoes, garlic and spring onions and cook for 2–3 minutes, stirring frequently.
- Add the basil, bay leaf, stock and tomato purée.
- Season with freshly ground black pepper but do not add further salt at this stage as the soup may be quite salty.

continued overleaf

- Bring to the boil and simmer for 20–30 minutes, then sieve the mixture into a clean saucepan.
- Mix the cornflour and a little cold water to make a smooth paste and add to the soup, mixing evenly. Stir over a low heat until the soup thickens.
- Add salt to taste, stir in the cream and serve garnished with chopped basil.

Carbohydrate content per serving: 20 grams

Chilled cucumber soup (FOR 2)

1 large cucumber, peeled and diced
400 ml vegetable stock
1½ tbsp chopped fresh chives
Pinch of sea salt
Freshly ground black pepper
100 ml single cream

- Add the cucumber to the stock in a large saucepan, bring to the boil then reduce the heat and simmer gently for 30 minutes.
- Stir in 1 tbsp of chives, season to taste and purée in a blender.
- Return the puréed soup to the pan, stir in the cream and heat through gently for about 3–4 minutes.
- Chill in the fridge for 2 hours then serve, garnished with the remaining chopped chives.

Carbohydrate content per serving: 16 grams

Carrot and orange soup

1 tbsp extra-virgin olive oil
1 medium red onion, peeled and finely chopped
1 medium red pepper, peeled, deseeded and chopped
300 grams carrots, peeled and sliced
400 ml Swiss bouillon stock
2 slices fresh root ginger, peeled and finely chopped
Juice of 1 freshly squeezed Seville orange
1 tbsp fresh coriander leaves, finely chopped (optional)
Freshly ground black pepper
2 tbsp crème fraîche

- Heat the olive oil in a medium saucepan and sauté the onion for 3–4 minutes.
- Add the red pepper, carrots, stock and ginger.
- Bring to the boil then simmer gently for about 25–30 minutes.
- Remove the pan from the heat and stir in the orange juice and coriander, if desired.
- Purée the soup in a blender.
- Return the soup to the pan and heat through gently.
- Season to taste and serve immediately, with a swirl of crème fraîche in each bowl.

Carbohydrate content per serving: 23 grams

Butternut squash and coriander soup (FOR 2)

2 tbsp extra-virgin olive oil
1 medium onion, peeled and diced
750 grams butternut squash, peeled and chopped
1½ tsp ground cumin
½ tsp ground turmeric
400 ml chicken stock
1 tbsp chopped fresh coriander
2 slices fresh root ginger, peeled and chopped finely
Pinch of rock salt
Freshly ground black pepper
100 ml single cream
1 tbsp chopped fresh chives

- Heat the olive oil in a large saucepan and sauté the onion and squash for 2–3 minutes.
- Stir in the cumin and turmeric and sauté for a further 2 minutes.
- Add the chicken stock, coriander and ginger, bring to the boil and simmer for 20–25 minutes.
- Transfer to a blender and purée then return the soup to the saucepan.
- Season to taste, stir in 80 ml of the cream and heat gently. Do not boil!
- Serve immediately with a swirl of cream and garnish with freshly chopped chives.

Carbohydrate content per serving: 15 grams

Creamy mushroom soup (FOR 2)

1 tbsp extra-virgin olive oil
2 shallots, peeled and finely chopped
1 garlic clove, peeled and finely chopped
60 grams button mushrooms, wiped and finely sliced
½ tbsp plain flour
200 ml chicken or vegetable stock
150 ml full-cream milk
Pinch of rock salt
Freshly ground black pepper
1 tbsp medium sherry (or Marsala)
1 tbsp freshly chopped flat-leaf parsley, to garnish

- Heat the olive oil in a medium saucepan and gently sauté the shallots and garlic for 2–3 minutes. Stir in the mushrooms and cook for a further 2–3 minutes.
- Remove from the heat and stir in the flour.
- Return to a gentle heat and stir in the stock and milk.
- Season to taste and simmer gently for 2–3 minutes, but do not allow to boil.
- Purée the soup in a blender.
- Stir in the sherry (or Marsala) and serve immediately, garnished with freshly chopped flat-leaf parsley.

Carbohydrate content per serving: 12 grams

Tofu and red pepper soup (FOR 2)

450 ml Swiss bouillon vegetable stock
2 slices fresh root ginger, peeled and grated
100 grams tofu, chopped into 2 cm cubes
1 small red pepper, deseeded and finely sliced
50 grams bamboo shoots, drained and finely sliced
2 spring onions, chopped diagonally into 1–2 cm lengths
Pinch of sea salt
Freshly ground black pepper
½ tbsp freshly chopped coriander leaves

- Bring the vegetable stock to the boil then add the ginger, tofu, red pepper, bamboo shoots and spring onions.
- Season to taste and simmer gently for 15 minutes.
- Serve immediately, sprinkled with chopped coriander.

Carbohydrate content per serving: 11 grams

Red pepper and basil soup (FOR 2)

1 tbsp extra-virgin olive oil
1 medium red onion, peeled and finely chopped
1 medium garlic clove, peeled and finely chopped
2 slices fresh root ginger, peeled and finely chopped
2 large red peppers, deseeded and sliced
200 grams tomatoes, peeled (see page 123) and chopped
400 ml Swiss bouillon vegetable stock
1 tbsp chopped fresh basil leaves
Freshly ground black pepper
1 tbsp crème fraîche

- Heat the oil in a medium saucepan and sauté the onion, garlic, ginger and peppers for 3–4 minutes.
- Add the tomatoes and vegetable stock to the pepper mixture, and simmer for 25–30 minutes.
- Purée the soup in a blender.
- Return the soup to the saucepan, stir in the basil and heat through gently.
- Season to taste and serve immediately, stirring ½ tbsp crème fraîche into each bowl.

Carbohydrate content per serving: 11 grams

Garden pea soup (FOR 2)

1 tbsp extra-virgin olive oil
3 shallots, peeled and diced
1 small leek, peeled and sliced
100 grams freshly shelled garden peas
1 medium potato, peeled and diced
400 ml Swiss bouillon vegetable stock
Freshly ground black pepper
1 tbsp freshly chopped basil leaves
Freshly chopped chives, to garnish

- Heat the olive oil in a large saucepan and sauté the shallots and leek for 4–5 minutes.
- Add the peas, potato and stock, season with black pepper, bring to the boil and simmer for 25–30 minutes.
- Purée the soup in a blender.
- Return the soup to the saucepan, stir in the basil and reheat gently.
- Serve immediately, garnished with chopped fresh chives.

Carbohydrate content per serving: 16 grams

Watercress soup (FOR 2)

25 grams butter
1 small onion, peeled and diced
150 grams watercress, finely chopped
250 ml chicken stock
150 ml full-cream milk
Pinch of rock salt
Freshly ground black pepper
1 tbsp freshly grated Parmesan cheese
1 tbsp fresh single cream

■ Melt the butter in a medium saucepan and gently sauté the onion for 3–4 minutes.
■ Stir in the watercress, cook for 2–3 minutes and then stir in the stock and milk.
■ Heat through and season to taste.
■ Gently simmer for 8–10 minutes.
■ Stir in the Parmesan cheese.
■ Remove from the heat and purée the soup in a blender.
■ Serve with a swirl of single cream.

Carbohydrate content per serving: 9 grams

Miso fish soup   (FOR 2)

500 ml Swiss bouillon vegetable stock
3 slices fresh root ginger, peeled and finely chopped
50 grams mangetout, top-and-tailed
1 medium red pepper, deseeded and finely sliced
2 spring onions, chopped into 3 cm lengths
1 tbsp mirin (Japanese sweet wine)
1 large green chilli, deseeded and finely chopped
100 grams fresh salmon fillets, chopped into 3 cm blocks
100 grams fresh cod fillets, chopped into 3 cm blocks
50 grams raw tiger prawns, peeled
1 tbsp miso paste
1 tbsp Shoyu (Japanese soy sauce)

- Add the stock, ginger, mangetout, pepper, spring onions, mirin and chilli to a large saucepan, bring to the boil and simmer gently for 8–10 minutes.
- Stir in the fish, prawns and miso paste and simmer for a further 4–5 minutes.
- Spoon into individual bowls and drizzle over a little Shoyu.

Carbohydrate content per serving: 9 grams

Char-grilled veggie soup (FOR 4)

500 grams firm ripe tomatoes, halved
1 medium red pepper, deseeded and sliced
1 medium green pepper, deseeded and sliced
1 garlic clove, peeled and finely chopped
3 slices fresh root ginger, peeled and chopped
1 medium red onion, peeled and quartered
1 medium green chilli, deseeded and chopped
2 tbsp extra-virgin olive oil
800 ml Swiss bouillon vegetable stock
1 tsp muscovado sugar
2 tbsp freshly squeezed lemon juice
Freshly ground black pepper

- Arrange the tomatoes, peppers, garlic, ginger, onion and chilli on a lined roasting tin, drizzle over the oil and cook at 180°C (gas mark 4) for 45–60 minutes.
- Transfer the vegetables to a blender, add the stock and blend until smooth.
- Stir in the sugar and lemon juice and season to taste.
- Transfer the mixture to a medium saucepan and heat through gently.
- Serve immediately.

Carbohydrate content per serving: 22 grams

Spicy chicken curry soup (FOR 2)

2 medium chicken breasts, skin removed
    (125–150 grams each)
30 grams butter
2 tbsp extra-virgin olive oil
1 medium red onion, peeled and diced
1 level tbsp plain flour
2 level tbsp medium curry powder
2 slices fresh root ginger, peeled and finely chopped
½ tsp cinnamon
1 large carrot, peeled and grated
600 ml chicken stock
50 ml crème fraîche

- Place the chicken breasts in a medium ovenproof dish, dot with butter, cover with pierced aluminium foil and cook in the centre of a preheated oven at 180°C (gas mark 4) for 20–25 minutes.
- Remove the chicken from the oven, allow to cool then chop into 3–4 cm cubes.
- Heat the olive oil in a large frying pan and sauté the onion for 3–4 minutes.
- Stir in the flour, curry powder, ginger, cinnamon and carrot.
- Gradually stir in the chicken stock.
- Add the chopped chicken to the pan and simmer gently for about 30 minutes.
- Stir in the crème fraîche and heat through gently for 1 minute. Serve immediately.

Carbohydrate content per serving: 15 grams

Chapter 10 Salads

Rocket and tofu salad (FOR 2)

1 tbsp sesame seeds
100 grams rocket leaves
100 grams tofu, chopped into small cubes
1 small red pepper, deseeded and sliced thinly
1 small yellow pepper, deseeded and sliced thinly
75 ml lemon vinaigrette (page 222)
Freshly ground black pepper
Sprigs of fresh mint, to garnish (optional)

- Place the sesame seeds in a small frying pan and dry-roast for 1–2 minutes.
- Mix together the sesame seeds, rocket, tofu and peppers in a medium salad bowl.
- Drizzle over the lemon vinaigrette and season to taste with black pepper.
- Garnish with sprigs of fresh mint, if desired.

Carbohydrate content per serving: 6 grams

Fennel and tomato salad (FOR 2)

2 fennel bulbs, trimmed, outer leaves removed and
    quartered lengthways
50 grams mangetout
4 spring onions, chopped finely
4 semi-dried (page 218) or sun-dried tomatoes, quartered
1 tbsp chopped fresh coriander
Freshly ground black pepper
50 grams rocket
Fresh shavings of Parmesan cheese and fresh basil
    leaves, to garnish

- Lightly steam the quartered fennel bulbs and
  mangetout, and set aside to cool.
- Mix together the fennel, mangetout, spring onions,
  tomatoes and coriander.
- Season to taste and serve on a bed of rocket.
- Garnish with fresh shavings of Parmesan cheese and
  basil leaves.

Carbohydrate content per serving: 12 grams

Caper and olive salad (FOR 2)

75 grams baby spinach leaves
2 spring onions, chopped into 2–3 cm pieces
2 large plum tomatoes, deseeded and chopped
1 tsp capers, rinsed
4–5 green olives, stoned and halved
4–5 black olives, stoned and halved
1 garlic clove, peeled and grated
25 grams pine nuts, lightly toasted
2 tsp chopped fresh basil
Pinch of rock salt
Freshly ground black pepper
Lemon vinaigrette (page 222)

- Mix together the baby spinach leaves, spring onions, tomatoes, capers, olives, garlic, pine nuts and basil.
- Season to taste and drizzle over the lemon vinaigrette.

Carbohydrate content per serving: 8 grams

Bocconcini and Parmesan salad   (FOR 2)

2 tomato vines, each with 6 cherry tomatoes
2 tbsp extra-virgin olive oil
75 grams wild rocket
75 grams Bocconcini cheese, sliced thinly
50 grams freshly grated Parmesan cheese
1 small Hass avocado, halved, peeled, stoned and
     chopped
1 tbsp chopped fresh basil leaves
1 tsp chopped fresh coriander leaves
Freshly ground black pepper
Balsamic vinaigrette (page 222)
Fresh basil leaves, to garnish

- Brush the cherry tomatoes (on the vine) with the olive
  oil and grill, 8 cm from the heat, for 2 minutes.
- Mix together the rocket, Bocconcini, Parmesan,
  avocado, basil and coriander. Season to taste.
- Place the warm cherry tomatoes (still on the vine) on
  the salad, and drizzle over the balsamic vinaigrette.
- Garnish with fresh basil leaves.

Carbohydrate content per serving: 4 grams

Green salad (FOR 2)

100 grams mixed crispy lettuce leaves (cos, curly endive,
coral, green oak leaf, mizuna)
1 medium Lebanese cucumber, sliced lengthways
1 celery stick, chopped diagonally
1 small green pepper, deseeded and sliced thinly
1 small ripe Hass avocado, halved, stoned and diced
Fresh basil leaves, to garnish

Dressing
4 tbsp extra-virgin olive oil
1 tbsp white wine vinegar
Freshly ground black pepper
Pinch of sugar
1 tsp Dijon mustard

■   Add the dressing ingredients to a screw-top jar and
    mix well.
■   Toss the salad ingredients in a large salad bowl and
    pour over the dressing. Garnish with fresh basil.

Carbohydrate content per serving: 6 grams

Red lettuce salad   FOR 2

100 grams mixed red lettuce leaves (radicchio, red oak
        lettuce, lollo rosso, mignonette)
1 small red pepper, deseeded and sliced thinly
1 red onion, peeled and sliced thinly
4 semi-dried tomatoes (page 218)
½ small red chilli, deseeded and chopped finely

■   Mix together the salad ingredients and drizzle over
    your choice of dressing.

Carbohydrate content per serving: 11 grams

Fennel and herb salad   FOR 2

1 bulb Florence fennel, washed and chopped
1 spring onion, chopped diagonally into 2–3 cm lengths
50 grams mangetout, topped and tailed
75 grams fresh watercress
1 tbsp chopped fresh basil
1 tbsp chopped fresh chives
Freshly ground black pepper
French vinaigrette (page 221)

■   Toss together the salad ingredients, season to taste
    with black pepper and drizzle over a little vinaigrette.
■   Serve immediately.

Carbohydrate content per serving: 8 grams

English cucumber with garden-fresh mint (FOR 2)

½ English cucumber, sliced very finely
2 tbsp natural yoghurt
1 tsp chopped fresh mint
1 tbsp freshly squeezed lime juice
Sprig of fresh mint, to garnish

- Place the cucumber slices in a colander and allow to drain for 10 minutes.

At the same time:

- Mix together the yoghurt, mint and lime juice.
- Place the cucumber slices on a plate, top with the yoghurt and garnish with a sprig of fresh mint.

Carbohydrate content per serving: 6 grams

Calamari salad   (FOR 2)

1 medium carrot
100 grams mixed salad leaves, such as ruby chard,
        watercress, spinach, lollo rosso
1 tbsp extra-virgin olive oil
150 grams calamari, sliced into medium rings
2 tbsp balsamic vinaigrette (page 222)
Fresh basil leaves, to garnish

- Peel the carrot and shave thinly.
- Mix the carrot shavings with the salad leaves.
- Heat the olive oil in a medium frying pan and stir-fry
  the calamari for 3–4 minutes.
- Arrange the calamari on a bed of salad leaves and
  drizzle over the dressing.
- Garnish with fresh basil leaves and serve immediately.

Carbohydrate content per serving: 5 grams

Watercress, spinach and avocado salad (FOR 2)

50 grams each baby spinach and watercress, washed
1 Lebanese cucumber, sliced vertically into thin slices
1 large ripe Hass avocado, peeled, stoned and sliced thinly
Juice of 1 freshly squeezed lime
2 tbsp French vinaigrette (page 221)

- Mix together the spinach, watercress, cucumber and avocado in a medium mixing bowl and drizzle over the lime juice.
- Drizzle over the dressing and serve immediately.

Carbohydrate content per serving: 4 grams

Mangetout and pistachio salad (FOR 2)

50 grams mangetout, topped and tailed
50 grams chickpeas, drained and rinsed
1 tbsp chopped fresh mint leaves
25 grams pistachio nuts, shells removed
French vinaigrette (page 221)
Freshly ground black pepper

- Lightly steam the mangetout for 3–4 minutes.
- Mix together the mangetout, chickpeas, mint leaves and pistachios in a medium mixing bowl.
- Drizzle over the dressing, season and serve.

Carbohydrate content per serving: 6 grams

Warm beef salad

300 grams sirloin steak, sliced thinly
2 tbsp extra-virgin olive oil
50 grams mangetout, topped and tailed
1 medium red pepper, deseeded and finely sliced
50 grams button mushrooms, wiped and halved
50 grams baby spinach leaves
3 slices fresh root ginger, peeled and finely sliced
1 tbsp chopped fresh coriander
Freshly ground black pepper

Marinade
Juice of 1 medium orange
1 medium garlic clove, peeled and chopped finely
1 tsp honey
1 tbsp hoi sin sauce
1 tbsp rice vinegar

- Combine the marinade ingredients in a medium mixing bowl and stir in the slices of steak.
- Chill for at least 1 hour in the fridge.
- Heat the olive oil in a wok and stir-fry the steak for 2–3 minutes.
- Add the mangetout, pepper, mushrooms, spinach and ginger and stir for a further 3–4 minutes.
- Stir in the coriander and stir-fry for a further minute then serve immediately, seasoned to taste.

Carbohydrate content per serving: 11 grams

Orange and berry salad   (FOR 2)

50 grams watercress
50 grams mixed green lettuce leaves
1 large Seville orange, peeled and sliced
50 grams strawberries, washed and sliced
50 grams blueberries, washed
50 grams raspberries, washed
1 medium Hass avocado, peeled, stoned and sliced
Freshly ground black pepper
Lemon vinaigrette (page 222)

- Add the watercress, lettuce leaves, orange, strawberries, blueberries, raspberries and avocado to a large serving bowl.
- Season to taste.
- Drizzle over the dressing and serve immediately.

Carbohydrate content per serving: 15 grams

Green salad with herbs   (FOR 2)

150 grams mixed green salad leaves, such as rocket,
    watercress, dandelion, baby spinach and fresh
    borage leaves
2 tsp chopped fresh basil
2 tsp chopped fresh coriander
2 tsp chopped fresh chervil
Pinch of rock salt
Freshly ground black pepper
French vinaigrette (page 221)

- Mix together the green salad leaves, basil, coriander
  and chervil, and season to taste.
- Drizzle over the French vinaigrette.

Carbohydrate content per serving: 2 grams

Rocket and olive salad   (FOR 2)

100 grams rocket leaves, washed
2 tsp capers, rinsed
50 grams black olives
3 anchovy fillets, chopped
1 tbsp chopped fresh coriander
1 tbsp freshly squeezed lemon juice
Freshly ground black pepper
60 ml balsamic vinaigrette (page 222)

- Mix together the rocket, capers, olives, anchovies, coriander and lemon juice, and season to taste.
- Drizzle over the balsamic vinaigrette.

Carbohydrate content per serving: 1 gram

Mozzarella and olive salad   (FOR 2)

75 grams mozzarella cheese, finely sliced
12 black olives, stoned and halved
1 Lebanese cucumber, chopped into cubes
1 tbsp fresh basil leaves, washed
Freshly ground black pepper

- Toss the ingredients of the salad and season to taste.

Carbohydrate content per serving: 4 grams

Chapter 11 Meat

Barbecue Thai lamb (FOR 2)

2 tsp garam masala
½ tsp ground cumin
½ tsp ground turmeric
1 small onion, peeled and chopped finely
1 garlic clove, peeled and chopped finely
3 slices of fresh root ginger, peeled and chopped finely
2 sticks of lemon grass, outer leaf discarded, chopped
    finely
1 tbsp chopped fresh coriander
1 tbsp Thai fish sauce
100 ml coconut milk
250 grams lean lamb fillet, cubed
Fresh coriander leaves, to garnish
Crispy green salad

- Add the garam masala, cumin and turmeric to a medium pan and dry stir-fry for about a minute.
- Transfer the spices to a food processor, add the onion, garlic, ginger, lemon grass, coriander, fish sauce and coconut milk and blend until smooth.

- Pour the marinade over the lamb, and marinate in the fridge for 3–4 hours.
- Soak some wooden skewers in water.
- Thread the lamb on to the skewers, and barbecue (or grill) for 6–8 minutes, turning frequently.
- Garnish with fresh coriander leaves, and serve immediately with a crispy green salad.

Carbohydrate content per serving: 10 grams

Lamb with basil sour cream   (FOR 2)

300 grams lean lamb fillet, cubed
Chopped fresh chives and sprigs of rosemary, to garnish
Crispy green salad

Marinade
3 tbsp extra-virgin olive oil
1 tbsp sweet sherry
1 garlic clove, peeled and grated finely
2 sprigs of fresh rosemary
2 tsp freshly squeezed lemon juice
Pinch of rock salt
Freshly ground black pepper

Basil sour cream
150 ml sour cream
1 tbsp chopped fresh basil
2 tsp chopped fresh chives

- Combine the marinade ingredients and marinate the lamb for 4–6 hours in the fridge.
- Soak wooden skewers for 2–3 hours before use.
- Mix together the sour cream, basil and chives, cover and cool in the fridge.
- Thread the meat on to the skewers and cook under a hot grill for 6–8 minutes, turning frequently.
- Pour the basil sour cream over the lamb skewers, garnish with chopped chives and fresh sprigs of rosemary, and serve with green salad (page 139).

Carbohydrate content per serving: 12 grams

Stir-fried lamb with oyster sauce (FOR 2)

3 tbsp extra-virgin olive oil
1 tsp sesame oil
200 grams lean lamb fillet, sliced finely
4 spring onions, chopped into 3–4 cm lengths
1 garlic clove, peeled and chopped finely
2 slices of fresh root ginger, peeled and chopped finely
1 small red pepper, deseeded and sliced finely
1 small yellow pepper, deseeded and sliced finely
1 small green pepper, deseeded and sliced finely
1 tbsp oyster sauce
2 tbsp sweet sherry
Freshly ground black pepper
Finely chopped spring onion, to garnish

- Heat 2 tbsp of olive oil and the sesame oil in a wok and stir-fry the lamb for 2–3 minutes, remove with a perforated spoon, set aside and cover.
- Heat the remaining olive oil in the wok and add the spring onions, garlic, ginger and peppers.
- Stir-fry for about 2 minutes then stir in the oyster sauce and sweet sherry.
- Season to taste, return the lamb to the wok and stir-fry for a final 2 minutes.
- Serve immediately, garnished with finely chopped spring onion.

Carbohydrate content per serving: 11 grams

Lamb with bok choi　(FOR 2)

3 tbsp extra-virgin olive oil
200 grams lean lamb, sliced into thin strips
1 tsp sesame oil
1 red onion, peeled and sliced finely
1 garlic clove, peeled and sliced finely
2 slices of fresh root ginger, peeled and chopped finely
1 small yellow pepper, deseeded and sliced
1 small red pepper, deseeded and sliced
1 tbsp each oyster sauce and light soy sauce
2 tbsp dry sherry
1 tsp caster sugar
Pinch of rock salt
Freshly ground black pepper
½ a bok choi (approximately 200 grams), shredded
Fresh coriander leaves, to garnish

- Heat 2 tbsp of olive oil in a wok and stir-fry the lamb
  for 3–4 minutes.
- Remove from the wok with a perforated spoon, cover
  and set aside.
- Heat the remaining olive oil and sesame oil in the
  wok, and sauté the onion and garlic for 1–2 minutes.
- Add the ginger, peppers, oyster sauce, soy sauce,
  sherry and sugar. Season to taste.
- Stir-fry for 2–3 minutes then add the bok choi, return
  the lamb to the wok and cook for a further 3 minutes
  on medium heat.
- Serve immediately, garnished with coriander leaves.

Carbohydrate content per serving: 12 grams

Beef korma

350 grams lean beef, cubed
4 tbsp extra-virgin olive oil
½ medium red onion, peeled and sliced
1 tbsp tomato purée
100 ml beef stock
Freshly ground black pepper
50 ml natural yoghurt
50 ml single cream
25 grams raw, unsalted cashew nuts
Fresh coriander leaves, to garnish
Green salad with herbs (page 146)

Marinade
1 medium red onion, peeled and diced finely
1 garlic clove, peeled and chopped finely
½ tsp cardamom seeds
1 tsp ground cumin
1 tsp ground coriander
2 slices of fresh root ginger, peeled and chopped finely
Pinch of cayenne pepper

- Add the ingredients of the marinade to a pestle, and grind to a paste.
- Brush the beef with 2 tbsp of extra-virgin olive oil.
- Coat the beef with the spice mixture, and marinate for 2–3 hours.
- Heat the remaining olive oil in a large frying pan and sauté the onion for 2–3 minutes.

continued overleaf

- Add the beef and cook over a low heat for 7–8 minutes, then stir in the tomato purée and stock.
- Simmer gently for 40–45 minutes, season to taste and stir in the yoghurt, cream and cashew nuts.
- Heat through gently, garnish with fresh coriander leaves and serve with green salad with herbs.

Carbohydrate content per serving: 12 grams

Beefburgers with herbs   (FOR 2)

250 grams lean minced beef (or lamb, pork or turkey)
1 small red onion, diced finely
1 small garlic clove, chopped finely
1 tbsp chopped fresh basil
1 tsp chopped fresh coriander
1 tsp Worcester sauce
1 medium free-range egg, beaten
Pinch of rock salt
Freshly ground black pepper
2 tbsp extra-virgin olive oil
Green salad with herbs (page 146)

- Mix together the mince, onion, garlic, basil, coriander, Worcester sauce and egg in a large mixing bowl, preferably by hand (definitely the best way to make hamburgers). Season to taste.
- Divide into 4 roughly equal pieces, then roll each into a ball and pat gently to flatten slightly.
- Chill in the fridge for 1–2 hours.
- Heat the olive oil in a medium frying pan, and cook the hamburgers for about 8 minutes (according to individual taste), turning once.
- Serve immediately with green salad and herbs.

Carbohydrate content per serving: 2 grams (without salad); 3 grams (with salad)

Steak and onions

3 tbsp extra-virgin olive oil
2 portions of frying steak (rump, sirloin or fillet,
        approximately 150 grams each)
1 medium brown onion, peeled and sliced thinly
1 medium red onion, peeled and sliced thinly
1 garlic clove, peeled and chopped finely
75 grams button mushrooms, wiped and sliced
Pinch of rock salt
Freshly ground black pepper
75 grams French beans

- Heat the olive oil in a medium frying pan and sear the steaks over a high heat. Add the onions and garlic, lower the heat and cook to taste: 3–4 minutes for rare, 4–6 minutes for medium and 6–8 minutes for well done. Cooking time depends on the heat of the pan and the thickness of the steaks.
- After 2–3 minutes, add the mushrooms and season to taste.
- As the steaks are cooking, lightly steam the French beans, and serve immediately.

Carbohydrate content per serving: 7 grams

Sesame beef with ginger and lemon grass (FOR 2)

If you are short of time you could try the quick method that follows this recipe.

4 tbsp extra-virgin olive oil
250 grams minute steak, sliced into strips
4 slices of fresh root ginger, peeled and chopped
2 stalks of lemon grass, husks removed, chopped finely
1 tbsp sesame seeds
75 grams carrot, peeled and sliced into julienne strips
75 grams mangetout
1 small red chilli, deseeded and chopped finely
1 medium red pepper, deseeded and sliced finely
1 tbsp chopped fresh chives, to garnish

- Heat 2 tbsp of the olive oil in a medium frying pan and gently stir-fry the minute steak for 2–3 minutes.
- Add the ginger, lemon grass and sesame seeds and stir-fry for a further 3–4 minutes.

At the same time:

- Heat the remaining 2 tbsp of olive oil in a wok and stir-fry the carrot, mangetout, chilli and pepper for 3–4 minutes.
- Serve the sesame beef with the vegetables, garnished with chopped chives.

Carbohydrate content per serving: 9 grams

Quick method

4 tbsp extra-virgin olive oil

250 grams minute steak, sliced into strips

4 slices of fresh root ginger, peeled and chopped

1 tbsp sesame seeds

2 tbsp Sharwoods sweet chilli and lemon grass sauce

300-gram packet of mixed stir-fry vegetables

1 tbsp chopped fresh chives, to garnish

- Heat 2 tbsp of the olive oil in a medium frying pan and gently fry the minute steak, ginger and sesame seeds for 3–4 minutes.
- Add the sweet chilli and lemon grass sauce and simmer gently for a further 3–4 minutes.

At the same time:

- Heat the remaining 2 tbsp of olive oil in a wok and stir-fry the vegetables for 2–3 minutes.
- Serve the sesame beef with the vegetables, garnished with chopped chives.

Carbohydrate content per serving: 14 grams

Spicy beef with horseradish   (FOR 2)

2 tbsp extra-virgin olive oil
300 grams casserole beef, cubed
1 large red onion, peeled and sliced
1 medium garlic clove, peeled and finely chopped
75 grams button mushrooms, wiped and halved
1 tbsp plain flour
½ tsp medium curry powder
½ tsp granulated sugar
½ tsp ground ginger powder
5–6 drops Tabasco sauce
400 ml beef stock
1 tbsp horseradish
1 tbsp fresh basil leaves, chopped
1 tbsp fresh oregano, chopped
50 grams each mangetout and sugar snap peas

■ Preheat the oven to 170°C (gas mark 3).
■ Heat the olive oil in a medium frying pan and brown
   the beef cubes for 2–3 minutes.
■ Add the onion, garlic and mushrooms.
■ Stir in the flour, curry powder, sugar, ginger, Tabasco
   sauce and stock.
■ Transfer to a casserole dish, cover and cook in the
   centre of the oven for 1½ hours.
■ Stir in the horseradish, basil and oregano and cook
   for a further 20–30 minutes.
■ Steam the mangetout and sugar snap peas and serve
   with the spicy beef.

Carbohydrate content per serving: 17 grams

Roast ham with Leerdammer cheese and mustard (FOR 1)

30 grams (approximately) red lettuce salad leaves
    (radicchio, red oak lettuce, lollo rosso)
Drizzle of French vinaigrette (page 221)
2–3 slices of thick honey roast ham
1 slice of Leerdammer cheese (pre-sliced)
1 tsp wholegrain mustard
Freshly ground black pepper

- Arrange the salad leaves on a plate.
- Drizzle over a little French vinaigrette. This can be easily be made at home and stored for later use, or you can use a commercial variety.
- Top with the honey roast ham and Leerdammer cheese, with a tsp of delicious wholegrain mustard.
- Season to taste with black pepper.

Carbohydrate content per serving: 1 gram

Honey mustard ham and (FOR 2)
Camembert frittata

4 medium organic free-range eggs
1 tbsp chopped flat-leaf parsley
1 tbsp extra-virgin olive oil
150 grams honey mustard ham, finely chopped
50 grams Camembert cheese, finely sliced
Freshly ground black pepper

- Beat together the eggs and parsley.
- Heat the oil in a medium frying pan and add the egg mixture.
- Cook until the eggs just begin to set then sprinkle over the ham and Camembert.
- Cook under a preheated grill (no closer than 8–10 cm to the heat) for approximately 2 minutes until the cheese begins to brown.
- Season with black pepper and serve immediately.

Carbohydrate content per serving: 2 grams

Peppered smoked ham with spinach and ricotta (FOR 2)

½ tbsp sesame seeds (optional)
2 tbsp extra-virgin olive oil
75 grams baby spinach leaves
1 garlic clove, peeled and chopped finely
50 grams ricotta cheese, crumbled
Freshly ground black pepper
4 thick slices of pre-cooked peppered smoked ham

- If using the sesame seeds, dry stir-fry them in a medium frying pan (or wok) for 1 minute.
- Heat the olive oil in the pan (or wok) and stir-fry the spinach and garlic for about 1 minute.
- Stir in the ricotta cheese and cook for a further minute.
- Season to taste with black pepper and serve immediately with the peppered smoked ham.

Carbohydrate content per serving: 2 grams

Pancetta, lettuce and tomato open sandwich

4 rashers of pancetta (or lean bacon)
Small handful of mixed lettuce leaves (frisée, mizuna, green
      oak, rocket)
2 slices buttered wholemeal bread (or toast)
2 medium plum tomatoes (preferably on the vine), sliced
Drizzle of Worcester sauce (optional)
Freshly ground black pepper

- Grill the pancetta (or bacon).
- Arrange the mixed lettuce leaves on the buttered
  wholemeal bread (or toast).
- Top with tomato slices and cooked pancetta rashers.
- Drizzle over a few drops of Worcester sauce, if using,
  and season to taste with black pepper.

*Carbohydrate content per serving: 19 grams (only 2 grams without
bread)*

Pork chops with beetroot salsa (FOR 2)

2 medium lean pork chops (approximately 150 grams
    each)
100 ml red wine
1 tbsp balsamic vinegar
2 sprigs of rosemary
50 grams courgettes, sliced
50 grams mangetout, topped and tailed

Beetroot salsa
100 grams cooked beetroot, peeled and finely chopped
2 shallots, peeled and finely chopped
1 tbsp freshly grated horseradish

- Preheat the oven to 180°C (gas mark 4).
- Place the pork chops in a medium ovenproof dish,
  pour over the red wine and balsamic vinegar and
  place the sprigs of rosemary on top.
- Cover with pierced aluminium foil and cook in the
  centre of the oven for 25–30 minutes.

At the same time:

- Mix together the beetroot, shallots and horseradish
  then chill in the fridge.
- Just before the pork is ready, steam the courgettes
  and mangetout for about 5 minutes.
- Serve the pork with beetroot salsa, courgettes and
  mangetout.

Carbohydrate content per serving: 11 grams

Chapter 12   Poultry

Chicken and ginger   (FOR 2)

3 tbsp extra-virgin olive oil
2 skinless chicken breast fillets, thinly sliced diagonally
3 spring onions, chopped into 3–4 cm lengths
1 garlic clove, peeled and chopped finely
3 slices of fresh root ginger, peeled and chopped finely
75 grams mangetout
1 medium red pepper, deseeded and sliced finely
25 grams raw cashew nuts
1 tbsp light soy sauce
1 tbsp dry sherry
Freshly ground black pepper
2 tsp chopped fresh chives

- Heat 2 tbsp of the olive oil in a wok and stir-fry the chicken for 3–4 minutes.
- Remove with a perforated spoon and set aside.
- Heat the remaining tbsp of olive oil in the wok, and sauté the spring onions and garlic for 1–2 minutes.
- Add the ginger, mangetout, pepper, cashew nuts, soy sauce and sherry, and season to taste.

continued overleaf

- Stir-fry for 2–3 minutes then return the chicken to the wok and cook for a further 2–3 minutes.
- Serve immediately, garnished with chopped chives.

Carbohydrate content per serving: 12 grams

Chicken breast with chilli sauce   (FOR 1)

To save time, you can use a ready-cooked chicken breast.

1 chicken breast
25 grams unsalted butter, cubed
½ Lebanese cucumber, cubed
4 cherry tomatoes on the vine, halved
2 tsp chilli sauce
30 grams (approximately) rocket and watercress leaves
Freshly ground black pepper

- Preheat the oven to 180°C (gas mark 4).
- Place the chicken breast in an ovenproof dish and dot with cubes of butter.
- Cover with pierced aluminium foil and cook in the centre of the oven for 35–40 minutes, then set aside to cool.
- Slice the chicken breast and mix with the cucumber, tomatoes and chilli sauce in a medium bowl.
- Make a bed of rocket and watercress leaves on a plate and top with the chilli chicken mixture.
- Season to taste with freshly ground black pepper.

Carbohydrate content per serving: 4 grams

Lemon chicken

1 medium red onion, peeled and chopped
3 slices of fresh root ginger, peeled and finely chopped
1 tbsp chopped basil leaves
1 tbsp chopped flat-leaf parsley
1 tbsp Shoyu (Japanese soy sauce)
1 tbsp dry sherry
4 tbsp freshly squeezed lemon juice
Pinch of rock salt
Freshly ground black pepper
Medium fresh organic chicken (1.5 kg)
1 lime, sliced
2 tbsp extra-virgin olive oil
250 ml chicken stock

- Preheat the oven to 180°C (gas mark 4).
- Mix together the onion, ginger, basil, parsley, Shoyu, sherry and lemon juice, season to taste and blend until smooth.
- Loosen the skin under the chicken breast and slide the puréed mixture under the skin.
- Place the lime slices in the chicken cavity.
- Put the chicken in a roasting tin and brush with the olive oil. Pour the stock into the roasting tin.
- Cook the chicken allowing 20 minutes per 450 grams plus 20 minutes extra.
- Serve immediately with a green salad.

Carbohydrate content per serving: 22 grams

Breast of chicken with (FOR 2) savoury filling

2 medium organic chicken breasts with skin (about
      150 grams each)
50 grams butter, cubed
100 grams pumpkin, chopped into cubes
50 grams sugar snap peas
Freshly ground black pepper

Stuffing
30 grams butter
1 medium red onion, peeled and diced
1 large apple, peeled, cored and grated
25 grams freshly grated Parmesan cheese
25 grams fresh breadcrumbs
1 tbsp chopped fresh basil

- Preheat the oven to 180°C (gas mark 4).
- To start making the stuffing, melt the butter in a medium frying pan and sauté the onion for 2–3 minutes.
- Stir in the apple, Parmesan cheese, breadcrumbs and basil and sauté for 2–3 minutes.
- Loosen the chicken skin and pack the stuffing between the skin and the breasts, forming a thin layer.
- Place the chicken breasts in a medium roasting tin and dot with butter cubes.
- Place the pumpkin around the chicken breasts, cover with pierced aluminium foil and cook in the centre of the oven for about 45 minutes.

- 10 minutes before the chicken is ready, add the sugar snap peas to the tin.
- Serve the chicken with the pumpkin and sugar snap peas, seasoning to taste.

Carbohydrate content per serving: 21 grams

Citrus chicken kebabs　(FOR 2)

2 chicken breasts, skin removed and chopped into cubes
1 medium green pepper, deseeded and chopped into
　　chunks
1 medium yellow pepper, deseeded and chopped into
　　chunks
50 grams mushrooms, wiped and halved
Freshly ground black pepper

Marinade
Juice of 1 freshly squeezed lemon
Juice of 1 freshly squeezed lime
1 tbsp extra-virgin olive oil
3 slices of fresh root ginger, peeled and finely chopped
1 medium garlic clove, peeled and finely chopped

- Mix together the marinade ingredients in a medium
  mixing bowl.
- Stir in the chicken cubes and marinate for about
  45 minutes in the fridge. Meanwhile, soak some
  wooden skewers in water.
- Thread the chicken, peppers and mushrooms on to
  the skewers and pour over a little of the remaining
  citrus marinade.
- Grill for 15–20 minutes (no closer than 8–10 cm to
  the heat), turning frequently.
- Season to taste and serve immediately.

Carbohydrate content per serving: 10 grams

Poached chicken and leeks

2 medium chicken breasts (approximately 125–150 grams
        each), skin removed
100 ml chicken stock
50 ml dry vermouth
50 grams butter
2 large leeks, topped and tailed and chopped into rings
1 tbsp plain flour
1 tsp wholegrain mustard
1 tbsp chopped fresh flat-leaf parsley
Freshly ground black pepper

■   Place the chicken breasts in a medium frying pan, stir in
    the stock and vermouth, bring to the boil then lower the
    heat and poach the chicken for about 8–10 minutes.

At the same time:

■   Heat 25 grams of the butter in a medium saucepan,
    add the leeks and sauté gently for about 5 minutes.
■   With a slotted spoon, add the leeks to the chicken.
■   Mix together the remaining butter, flour and mustard in
    a small bowl.
■   Remove the chicken and leeks from the frying pan
    and gradually add the butter mixture to the pan,
    stirring constantly, until the sauce begins to thicken.
■   Return the leeks and chicken to the pan, stir in the
    parsley and heat through gently.
■   Season to taste and serve immediately.

Carbohydrate content per serving: 10 grams

Turkey and avocado

1 medium Hass avocado, halved, stoned, peeled and
    chopped finely
1 tbsp mayonnaise, commercial or home-made (page 220)
2 tsp freshly squeezed lemon juice
3 spring onions, chopped into 3–4 cm lengths
½ tbsp chopped fresh basil
Freshly ground black pepper
4 slices of cooked turkey breast
2 slices of buttered wholemeal toast (optional)
4 semi-dried tomatoes (page 218) or commercial sun-dried
    tomatoes
Sprigs of fresh basil, to garnish
Rocket and olive salad (page 147)

- Mix together the avocado, mayonnaise, lemon juice,
  spring onions, basil and black pepper in a small bowl.
- Place 2 slices of cooked turkey breast on each slice
  of toast (or directly on to the centre of the plate if you
  don't want an open sandwich).
- Spoon on the avocado mixture, and top with semi-
  dried or sun-dried tomatoes.
- Garnish with sprigs of fresh basil.
- Serve with rocket and olive salad.

*Carbohydrate content per serving: 26 grams (or 9 grams without
bread)*

Stir-fried turkey with cranberries (FOR 2)

50 grams fresh cranberries

2 tsp muscovado sugar

50 ml cranberry juice

50 ml orange juice

1 tbsp soy sauce

4 raw turkey breasts (approximately 200 grams each),
    sliced

2 tbsp extra-virgin olive oil

2 slices fresh root ginger, peeled and chopped

50 grams mangetout, top-and-tailed

50 grams sugar snap peas, top-and-tailed

50 grams button mushrooms, wiped and halved

- Place the cranberries and sugar in a wok with about 50 ml water.
- Bring to the boil and simmer for about 8–10 minutes.
- Remove from the wok and set aside.
- Add the cranberry juice, orange juice, soy sauce and turkey slices to a medium mixing bowl and marinate for 20 minutes.
- Heat the olive oil in a wok, drain the turkey with a slotted spoon and stir-fry for approximately 3–4 minutes.
- Stir in the ginger, mangetout, sugar snap peas and mushrooms, add 2 tbsp of the marinade and stir-fry for a further 3–4 minutes.
- Finally, stir in the cranberries and stir-fry for a final 2 minutes.
- Serve immediately.

Carbohydrate content per serving: 12 grams

Spicy turkey burgers (FOR 2)

250 grams turkey mince
2 slices fresh root ginger, peeled and finely chopped
1 medium garlic clove, peeled and finely chopped
1 tbsp soy sauce
1 tsp ground cumin
1 tbsp chopped fresh coriander leaves
1 tbsp chopped fresh flat-leaf parsley
1 large green chilli, deseeded and finely chopped
2 tbsp freshly squeezed lemon juice
2 lemon grass stalks, peeled and finely chopped
50 grams mangetout
1 medium red pepper, deseeded and finely sliced
Freshly ground black pepper

- Mix together the turkey mince, ginger, garlic, soy sauce, cumin, coriander, flat-leaf parsley, chilli, lemon juice and lemon grass in a large mixing bowl.
- Form the mixture into small even-sized burgers and flatten slightly.
- Cook under a medium grill (no closer than 8–10 cm to the heat) for about 8–10 minutes, turning once.

At the same time:

- Lightly steam the mangetout and pepper.
- Serve the turkey burgers with the mangetout and pepper and season to taste.

Carbohydrate content per serving: 8 grams

Stir-fried duck with vegetables (FOR 2)

2 tbsp extra-virgin olive oil
2 medium duck breasts (125–150 grams each), finely
     sliced
2 tbsp plum sauce
1 tsp hoi sin sauce
Few drops of sesame oil
1 small red chilli, deseeded and finely chopped
1 medium organic free-range egg, beaten
1 medium red pepper, deseeded and finely sliced
1 medium yellow pepper, deseeded and finely sliced
50 grams mangetout, topped and tailed
1 tbsp cornflour
Freshly ground black pepper

- Heat the olive oil in a wok and stir-fry the duck breast
  slices for 3–4 minutes.
- Stir in the plum sauce, hoi sin sauce, sesame oil,
  chilli, egg, peppers and mangetout.
- Stir in the cornflour and stir-fry for 7–8 minutes.
- Season to taste and serve immediately.

Carbohydrate content per serving: 16 grams

Peking duck (FOR 2)

2 tbsp dry sherry
1 tbsp liquid honey
1 tbsp light soy sauce
3 tbsp freshly squeezed orange juice (or packaged orange
    juice if necessary)
2 slices of fresh root ginger, peeled and grated
2 duck breasts (approximately 150 grams each)
Baby leeks in lemon butter sauce (page 219)
Freshly ground black pepper
2 spring onions sliced finely lengthways, to garnish

- Mix together the sherry, honey, soy sauce, orange juice
  and ginger, and marinate the duck breasts for as long
  as possible (at least 20 minutes). Ideally, plan ahead
  and marinate the duck breasts overnight in the fridge.
- Preheat the oven to 180°C (gas mark 4).
- Place the duck breasts on a rack in a roasting tin,
  pour over the remaining marinade and roast in the
  centre of the oven for 30–35 minutes.
- Remove the duck from the oven, allow to cool for
  10–15 minutes then carve into thin slices.

At the same time:

- Prepare the baby leeks in lemon butter sauce.
- Serve the duck breast slices on a bed of leeks,
  season to taste and garnish with chopped spring
  onions.

Carbohydrate content per serving: 10 grams

Breast of duck with baby spinach (FOR 2)

2 duck breasts (approximately 150 grams each), sliced
        into thin strips
2 tbsp extra-virgin olive oil
50 grams sugar snap peas, topped and tailed
50 grams French beans, topped and tailed
1 medium yellow pepper, deseeded and sliced finely
100 grams baby spinach leaves

Marinade
1 tbsp freshly squeezed orange juice
1 tbsp balsamic vinegar
1 tbsp dry sherry

- Mix together the ingredients for the marinade.
- Place the duck strips in a shallow dish, add the
  marinade and marinate in the refrigerator for about
  20–30 minutes.
- Drain the marinade into a separate dish.
- Heat the olive oil in a wok and stir-fry the duck for
  about 2–3 minutes.
- Add the sugar snap peas, French beans, yellow
  pepper and baby spinach leaves and stir-fry for a
  further 2 minutes.
- Stir in the marinade, stir-fry for a minute and serve
  immediately.

Carbohydrate content per serving: 9 grams

Ginger duck (FOR 2)

Juice of 1 freshly squeezed lime
1 stalk of lemon grass, trimmed and chopped
1 garlic clove, peeled and finely chopped
4 slices fresh root ginger, peeled and sliced
1 large green chilli, deseeded and chopped
1 tbsp fish sauce
2 duck breasts
1 tbsp extra-virgin olive oil
1 pak choi, halved
Freshly ground black pepper

- Preheat the oven to 180°C (gas mark 4).
- Add the lime juice, lemon grass, garlic, ginger, chilli and fish sauce to a blender and blend until smooth.
- Brush the mixture on to the duck breasts and place in an ovenproof baking dish. Brush over a little olive oil.
- Cover with pierced aluminium foil and bake in the centre of the oven for 25–30 minutes.

At the same time:

- Lightly steam the pak choi for about 4–5 minutes.
- Serve the duck with the pak choi and season to taste.

Carbohydrate content per serving: 4 grams

Chapter 13 Fish

Salmon steaks with leek and lemon butter sauce (FOR 2)

2 salmon steaks (125–150 grams each)
3 tbsp extra-virgin olive oil
Freshly ground black pepper
Sprigs of fresh dill, to garnish
Green salad (page 139)

Leek and lemon butter sauce
1 small leek, chopped into 1–2 cm segments
75 grams butter
2 tbsp freshly squeezed lemon juice
1 tbsp chopped fresh basil
Freshly ground black pepper

To make the sauce:

- Lightly steam the chopped leek for 4–5 minutes.
- Melt the butter in a medium saucepan, stir in the leek, lemon juice, chopped basil and black pepper.

continued overleaf

At the same time:

- Brush the salmon with olive oil on both sides and season with black pepper.
- Cook under a medium grill for 4–5 minutes each side.
- Pour over the leek and lemon butter sauce.
- Garnish with fresh dill, and serve with green salad.

Carbohydrate content per serving: 4 grams (including salad)

Salmon with rocket and mint sauce   (FOR 2)

Rocket and mint sauce (page 226)
2 salmon fillets (approximately 150 grams each)
Pinch of rock salt
Pinch of paprika

- Prepare the rocket and mint sauce.
- Preheat the oven to 180°C (gas mark 4).
- Place the salmon fillets in a shallow ovenproof dish (in a single layer), cover with pierced aluminium foil and cook in the centre of the oven for 15–20 minutes.
- Season with salt, to taste, and serve immediately with rocket and mint sauce, garnished with a pinch of paprika.

Carbohydrate content per serving: 2 grams (including sauce)

Teriyaki salmon kebabs (FOR 2)
with cucumber dip

2 medium salmon fillets
½ cucumber, halved lengthways, deseeded and finely sliced
2 tsp rice vinegar
50 grams wholegrain rice
A few sprigs of dill, to garnish
Freshly ground black pepper

Marinade
2 tbsp sake (Japanese rice wine)
2 tbsp mirin (Japanese sweet wine)
2 tbsp Shoyu (Japanese soy sauce, such as tamari)

- Mix together the marinade ingredients in a small bowl.
- Place the salmon fillets on a plate and pour over the marinade.
- Cook the salmon under a medium grill (no closer than 8–10 cm to the heat) for about 8 minutes, turning once.

At the same time:

- Mix together the cucumber and rice vinegar and separate into 2 small bowls.
- Cook the rice.
- Serve the salmon on a bed of rice, garnished with dill.
- Put a bowl of cucumber and rice vinegar on each plate.
- Season to taste with freshly ground black pepper.

Carbohydrate content per serving: 22 grams

Smoked salmon with fennel and dill (FOR 2)

100 grams smoked salmon, finely sliced
1 tbsp freshly squeezed lime juice
1 tbsp Parmesan shavings
Freshly ground black pepper

Sauce
75 ml crème fraîche
½ tbsp finely chopped fresh fennel
½ tbsp finely chopped fresh dill

- Place the smoked salmon strips in the centre of the plates.
- Drizzle over a little lime juice.
- Mix together the crème fraîche, fennel and dill and pour over the smoked salmon.
- Top with Parmesan shavings and season to taste with black pepper.

Carbohydrate content per serving: 3 grams

Smoked haddock soufflé (FOR 4)

100 grams smoked haddock
250 ml full-cream milk
1 bay leaf
3 large free-range eggs
25 grams butter
25 grams plain flour
1 tbsp chopped fresh basil
Pinch of rock salt
Freshly ground black pepper
1 tbsp chopped fresh dill, to garnish
Rocket and olive salad (page 147)

- Preheat the oven to 180°C (gas mark 4).
- Place the haddock in the base of a baking dish, pour 100 ml of milk around the fish and add the bay leaf.
- Cover with pierced aluminium foil and bake in the centre of the oven for 10–12 minutes.
- Remove the haddock with a draining spoon and allow to cool before flaking the fish.
- Increase the oven temperature to 200°C (gas mark 6).
- Separate the eggs. Beat the yolks and whisk the whites until thickened.
- Melt the butter in a small saucepan then stir in the flour, chopped basil and remaining 150 ml of milk, stirring constantly until the mixture is evenly thickened.
- Remove from the heat and allow to cool for a couple of minutes, stirring occasionally.

continued overleaf

- Season to taste, then stir in the egg yolks and flaked haddock.
- Gradually 'fold' the egg whites into the mixture.
- Lightly butter 4 individual soufflé dishes and gently spoon in the mixture evenly.
- Place the soufflé dishes on a baking tray and bake in the centre of the oven for 25–30 minutes. (Ovens vary; the deciding factor is whether the soufflé has risen and is lightly browned.)
- The soufflé must be served immediately or it will collapse!
- Garnish with chopped fresh dill and serve with rocket and olive salad.

Carbohydrate content per serving: 15 grams (including salad)

Taramasalata

1 thin slice of white bread, crust removed
2 tbsp full-cream milk
150 grams smoked cod roe, skin removed
½ garlic clove, peeled and chopped finely
½ small white onion, peeled and grated finely
3 tbsp extra-virgin olive oil
1 tbsp freshly squeezed lemon juice
Freshly ground black pepper
Chopped fresh chives, to garnish
Red lettuce salad (page 140)

- Soak the bread in the milk, drain through a sieve and chop finely.
- Stir in the cod roe, garlic and onion, then gradually mix in the olive oil.
- Add the lemon juice, and season to taste with black pepper (salt will probably not be necessary as cod roe is naturally salty).
- Blend until smooth and chill in the fridge for 3–4 hours before serving.
- Just before serving, garnish with chopped fresh chives and serve with red lettuce salad.

Carbohydrate content per serving: 11 grams (including salad)

Poached whiting with ginger (FOR 2)

4 medium whiting fillets (about 75 grams each)
8 baby leeks
Julienne strips of ginger and spring onion, to garnish

Sauce
100 ml full-cream milk
2 tbsp sweet sherry
1 tbsp light soy sauce
1 garlic clove, peeled and grated
2 slices of fresh root ginger, peeled and grated
Pinch of rock salt
Freshly ground black pepper
2 tsp freshly squeezed lemon juice

- Mix together the ingredients for the sauce.
- Place the fillets in a single layer in the base of a large frying pan, and pour over the sauce.
- Bring to the boil then reduce the heat to a gentle simmer for about 10–12 minutes.

Just before the whiting is ready:

- Lightly steam the baby leeks for 3–4 minutes.
- Serve the whiting (pouring any remaining sauce over the fish) with the baby leeks.
- Garnish with julienne ginger and spring onion.

Carbohydrate content per serving: 5 grams

Fresh trout with mustard mayonnaise (FOR 2)

2 large fresh trout fillets
25 grams butter, cubed
2 tbsp mustard mayonnaise (page 220)
1 tbsp freshly squeezed orange juice
Freshly ground black pepper
1 tbsp freshly chopped chives, to garnish

- Preheat the oven to 180°C (gas mark 4).
- Place the trout fillets in an ovenproof dish, dot with butter, cover with pierced aluminium foil and cook in the centre of the oven for 18–20 minutes.

At the same time:

- Prepare the mustard mayonnaise.
- Lay the trout fillets in the centre of the plates and drizzle over the orange juice.
- Spoon the mustard mayonnaise next to the trout, season to taste and garnish with freshly chopped chives.
- Serve immediately.

Carbohydrate content per serving: 2 grams

Char-grilled swordfish with mustard dressing (FOR 2)

2 medium swordfish steaks (approximately 150 grams
    each)
2 tbsp extra-virgin olive oil
1 pak choi, halved lengthways
Mustard vinaigrette (page 221)
Freshly ground black pepper

- Brush the swordfish steaks with olive oil and cook
  under a hot grill (no closer than 8–10 cm to the heat)
  for 6–8 minutes, turning once.

At the same time:

- Lightly steam the pak choi for 5–6 minutes (or
  microwave, in a microwave-safe container, for
  2–3 minutes).

And

- Prepare the mustard vinaigrette.
- Serve the swordfish steaks with the pak choi, drizzle
  over the mustard vinaigrette and season to taste.

Carbohydrate content per serving: 3 grams

Baked cod with herbs   (FOR 2)

2 cod steaks (approximately 150 grams each), skin and
    bones removed
1½ tbsp plain flour
Pinch of rock salt
Freshly ground black pepper
2 tbsp extra-virgin olive oil
1 medium red onion, peeled and sliced finely
1 garlic clove, peeled and chopped finely
75 grams button mushrooms, wiped and halved
1 medium yellow pepper, deseeded and sliced thinly
200-gram tin of plum tomatoes, chopped
1 tbsp chopped fresh basil
2 tsp chopped fresh coriander
100 grams broccoli florets

- Preheat the oven to 180°C (gas mark 4).
- Coat the cod steaks with seasoned flour.
- Heat the olive oil in a small frying pan and sear the cod.
- Transfer the cod to an ovenproof dish.
- Gently sauté the onion and garlic in the frying pan for
  about a minute, then add the mushrooms and pepper
  for a further 1–2 minutes.
- Transfer the vegetables to the ovenproof dish, stir in
  the tomatoes, basil and coriander, season to taste and
  cook in the centre of the oven for 30–35 minutes.
- Lightly steam the broccoli florets.
- Serve the casserole immediately with the broccoli
  florets.

Carbohydrate content per serving: 18 grams

Citrus cod and rocket (FOR 2)

300 grams cod fillet, chopped into 3–4 cm cubes
100 grams rocket
Lemon wedges

Marinade
Juice of ½ a freshly squeezed orange
Juice of ½ a freshly squeezed lime
1 tbsp sweet sherry
2 tbsp extra-virgin olive oil
1 slice of fresh root ginger, peeled and chopped finely
1 tsp chopped fresh mint
Freshly ground black pepper

- Prepare the marinade.
- Marinate the cod for 4–6 hours in the fridge and soak some wooden skewers in water.
- Thread the cod on to the skewers, and cook under a hot grill (or barbecue) for 6–8 minutes, turning and basting with the marinade frequently.
- Serve on a bed of fresh rocket, with lemon wedges.

Carbohydrate content per serving: 4 grams

Spicy salsa cod   (FOR 2)

2 medium cod steaks (approximately 150 grams each)
50 grams mangetout
1 tbsp chopped fresh chives, to garnish

Marinade

1 medium garlic clove, peeled and diced
1 tbsp freshly squeezed lemon juice
2 tsp sun-dried tomato paste
100 ml natural yoghurt
1 slice fresh root ginger, peeled and finely chopped

Salsa

100 grams cucumber, finely chopped
2 tbsp freshly squeezed lemon juice
1 small red chilli, deseeded and finely chopped
1 spring onion, trimmed and chopped into 3 cm lengths
150 grams plum tomatoes, chopped

- Add the garlic, lemon juice, tomato paste, yoghurt and ginger to a medium mixing bowl and stir thoroughly.
- Coat the cod on both sides with the marinade and chill in the fridge for 45–60 minutes.
- Mix together the cucumber, lemon juice, chilli, spring onion and tomatoes in a medium mixing bowl.
- Cook the cod steaks under a medium grill (no closer than 8–10 cm to the heat) for about 8–10 minutes, turning once. Steam the mangetout for 4 minutes.
- Serve the cod with the salsa, mangetout and chives.

Carbohydrate content per serving: 17 grams

Oven-baked mackerel with (FOR 2) herb butter

50 grams unsalted butter
1 tbsp chopped fresh basil
1 tbsp chopped fresh coriander
1 tbsp freshly squeezed lemon juice
2 large fresh mackerel, gutted and cleaned
Freshly ground black pepper
Rocket and olive salad (page 147)

- Preheat the oven to 180°C (gas mark 4).
- Heat the butter in a small saucepan until just melted then stir in the basil, coriander and lemon juice.
- Score the mackerel several times on one surface then pour the herb butter mixture into the cavity and scores along the fish.
- Season to taste with black pepper.
- Wrap loosely in aluminium foil and cook in the centre of the oven for 25–30 minutes.
- Serve immediately with rocket and olive salad.

Carbohydrate content per serving: 20 grams

Fillets of Dover sole with creamy mushroom sauce   (FOR 2)

2 Dover sole fillets (approximately 150 grams each)
100 ml dry white wine
20 grams unsalted butter
100 ml single cream
1 tsp cornflour
75 grams chestnut mushrooms, wiped and finely sliced
Freshly ground black pepper
Green salad (page 139)

- Preheat the oven to 180°C (gas mark 4).
- Place the sole in an ovenproof dish, pour over the wine, cover with pierced aluminium foil and cook in the centre of the oven for 20 minutes.
- Mix together the butter, cream and cornflour in a small bowl.
- When the sole has cooked, drain the liquid into a medium saucepan.
- Stir in the cornflour mixture and bring to the boil gently, stirring constantly.
- Add the mushrooms and cook for 1–2 minutes.
- Place the fish in the centre of the plates, pour over the mushroom sauce and season to taste.
- Serve with a crispy green salad.

Carbohydrate content per serving: 12 grams

Lemon sole with lime butter sauce (FOR 2)

1 egg yolk
2 tsp freshly squeezed lime juice
30 grams butter
2 tbsp extra-virgin olive oil
4 lemon sole fillets
50 grams sugar snap peas
30 ml crème fraîche
Freshly ground black pepper

- Mix together the egg yolk, 1 tsp of lime juice and about half the butter in a medium bowl.
- Place the bowl over a saucepan of steaming water.
- Whisk constantly until the mixture begins to thicken.
- Take the bowl from the heat and gradually stir in the remaining butter and lime juice.
- Heat the olive oil in a medium frying pan and cook the lemon sole for about 4 minutes, turning once.

At the same time:

- Steam the sugar snap peas for 3–4 minutes.
- Fold the crème fraîche into the sauce and season to taste.
- Serve the fish topped with the lime butter sauce, with the sugar snap peas on the side.

Carbohydrate content per serving: 3 grams

Grilled sardines with fennel and herb salad   (FOR 2)

4 large sardines, gutted and cleaned
2 tbsp extra-virgin olive oil
Fennel and herb salad (page 140)
Cucumber raita (page 224)
1 tbsp chopped fresh coriander leaves
1 tbsp chopped fresh chives
3 tbsp freshly squeezed lemon juice

- Place the sardines on a grill tray and brush with the olive oil.
- Grill the sardines for about 5–6 minutes each side, turning once, no closer than 8–10 cm to the heat.
- Serve the sardines with fennel and herb salad and cucumber raita, top with chopped fresh coriander and chives, and drizzle over the lemon juice.

Carbohydrate content per serving: 9 grams

Chapter 14 Shellfish

Chilli tiger prawns (FOR 2)

10 cooked tiger prawns
English cucumber with garden-fresh mint (page 141)
Lime wedges
Lime zest, to garnish

Marinade
1 garlic clove, peeled and grated
1 small red chilli, deseeded and chopped very finely
2 slices of fresh root ginger, peeled and chopped finely
2 tbsp light soy sauce
2 tbsp sweet sherry
2 tbsp extra-virgin olive oil
Juice of ½ a lemon, freshly squeezed
1 tsp sesame oil
Freshly ground black pepper

- Mix together the marinade ingredients in a medium-sized bowl.
- Shell the tiger prawns. The easiest way to shell a prawn is to remove the head and tail and break off the

legs. The shell will then peel easily. Be careful to remove all of the shell; it has an awful texture!

■ Marinate the prawns for 3–4 hours.

■ Grill or barbecue the prawns for 2–3 minutes, turning once and basting with the marinade.

■ Serve the chilli tiger prawns with cucumber and mint salad and lime wedges, garnished with lime zest.

Carbohydrate content per serving: 10 grams

Seared scallops with rocket salad (FOR 2)

2 tbsp extra-virgin olive oil
8 fresh medium scallops, corals removed
50 grams spinach
50 grams rocket
Balsamic vinaigrette (page 222)
Freshly ground black pepper
1 tbsp chopped fresh chives, to garnish

■ Heat the olive oil in a medium frying pan and cook the scallops for 4 minutes, turning once.

■ Lay the scallops on a bed of mixed spinach and rocket leaves and drizzle over a little balsamic vinaigrette.

■ Season to taste with black pepper, garnish with chopped chives and serve immediately.

Carbohydrate content per serving: 5 grams

Scallop and calamari salad   (FOR 2)

30 grams butter
4 large scallops
2 tbsp extra-virgin olive oil
1 tsp sesame oil
2 garlic cloves, peeled and chopped finely
2 slices of fresh root ginger, peeled and chopped finely
8 raw tiger prawns, peeled and de-veined (tails on)
200 grams fresh calamari tubes, chopped into 1 cm rings
100 grams mixed wild rocket and red oak lettuce
4 spring onions, chopped finely
1 tbsp chopped fresh coriander
Freshly ground black pepper
Oriental vinaigrette (page 223)
Lime wedges

- Melt the butter in a small saucepan.
- Separate the corals from the scallops, slice the scallops into rounds horizontally, and gently sauté the scallops (and corals) for 3–4 minutes. Remove from the pan with a perforated spoon, cover and set aside.
- Heat the olive oil and sesame oil in a wok and sauté the garlic and ginger for a minute. Add the prawns and calamari, and stir-fry for 2–3 minutes. Add the cooked scallops and heat through gently for about a minute.
- Toss the wild rocket, red oak lettuce, spring onions and coriander, season to taste and transfer to plates.
- Arrange the scallops, prawns and calamari on the salad, drizzle over the dressing and add lime wedges.

Carbohydrate content per serving: negligible

Calamari and scallops with flat mushrooms

2 tbsp extra-virgin olive oil

75 grams calamari, sliced into rings

6 large scallops (corals removed), sliced into horizontal
    rounds

6 raw tiger prawns, peeled

1 medium green chilli, deseeded and finely chopped

3 slices fresh root ginger, peeled and finely sliced

2 shallots, peeled and diced

4 large flat mushrooms, wiped and halved

1 tbsp Shoyu (Japanese soy sauce)

1 tbsp mirin (Japanese sweet wine)

1 tbsp chopped fresh coriander

A few drops of sesame oil

Freshly ground black pepper

Green salad (page139)

- Heat the olive oil in a wok and stir-fry the calamari,
  scallops and prawns for 4–5 minutes.
- Add the chilli, ginger and shallots and stir-fry for a
  further 2–3 minutes.
- Add the mushrooms, Shoyu, mirin and coriander,
  drizzle over a few drops of sesame oil and stir-fry for a
  further 1–2 minutes. Season with black pepper.
- Serve immediately with a crispy green salad.

Carbohydrate content per serving: 13 grams

Ginger scallops with rocket   (FOR 2)

4 slices of fresh root ginger, peeled and sliced into
 matchsticks
2 tbsp freshly squeezed lemon juice
2 spring onions, topped and tailed, sliced lengthways and
 chopped diagonally into 3 cm segments
8 fresh scallops, corals removed, sliced in half horizontally
2 tbsp extra-virgin olive oil
100 grams fresh rocket leaves
Basil leaves, to garnish
Freshly ground black pepper

- Mix together the ginger, lemon juice and spring onions
  and pour over the scallops in a medium mixing bowl.
- Chill in the fridge for at least 1 hour.
- Heat the olive oil in a medium frying pan and fry the
  scallops for 3–4 minutes, turning once.
- Place a bed of rocket on each plate, top with the
  scallops and drizzle over the remaining marinade.
- Garnish with fresh basil leaves and season with
  freshly ground black pepper.

Carbohydrate content per serving: 7 grams

Chapter 15 Vegetables

Stir-fried tofu with mushrooms ⟨ FOR 2 ⟩

150 grams tofu, chopped into 2 cm cubes
3 tbsp extra-virgin olive oil
75 grams mangetout
75 grams bamboo shoots, sliced into thin strips
75 grams button mushrooms, wiped and halved
2 slices fresh root ginger, peeled and finely chopped
1 tbsp sesame seeds
Freshly ground black pepper

Marinade
1 tsp granulated sugar
3 tbsp light soy sauce
3 tbsp dry sherry

- Rinse the chopped tofu and pat dry.
- Mix together the marinade ingredients and marinate the tofu for 6–8 hours.
- Heat 2 tbsp of the olive oil in a wok and stir-fry the tofu for 2–3 minutes, then remove from the wok with a perforated spoon and set aside.

continued overleaf

- Heat the remaining olive oil in the wok and stir-fry the mangetout, bamboo shoots, mushrooms and ginger for 2–3 minutes, then add the tofu and stir-fry for a final 2 minutes.

At the same time:

- Dry stir-fry the sesame seeds in a small saucepan for 1 minute.
- Season to taste and serve immediately, garnished with the toasted sesame seeds.

Carbohydrate content per serving: 14 grams

Fresh asparagus with lemon butter sauce   (FOR 2)

200 grams asparagus, washed and trimmed
75 grams butter
Juice of ½ a freshly squeezed lemon
Freshly ground black pepper
Fresh basil leaves, to garnish

- Lightly steam the asparagus.
- Melt the butter in a small saucepan, stir in the lemon juice and season to taste.
- Arrange the asparagus on warm plates, pour over the lemon butter sauce and garnish with fresh basil.

Carbohydrate content per serving: 4 grams

Bok choi with oyster sauce

2 tbsp extra-virgin olive oil
1 slice of fresh root ginger, peeled and chopped finely
1 bok choi, shredded
1 tbsp oyster sauce
Freshly ground black pepper
½ tsp sesame oil

- Heat the olive oil in a wok and sauté the ginger and bok choi for about a minute.
- Stir in the oyster sauce, season to taste and stir-fry for a further 2 minutes.
- Drizzle with sesame oil and serve immediately.

Carbohydrate content per serving: 3 grams

Broccoli with oyster sauce

Follow the recipe 'Bok choi with oyster sauce' (above), substituting the bok choi with 250 grams broccoli florets.

Carbohydrate content per serving: 3 grams

Char-grilled vegetables with (FOR 2) sesame seeds

1 tsp sesame seeds
1 small green pepper, deseeded and quartered lengthways
1 small red pepper, deseeded and quartered lengthways
2 small red onions, peeled and quartered lengthways
2 large plum tomatoes, quartered lengthways
4 yellow squash, halved lengthways
2 tbsp extra-virgin olive oil
Freshly ground black pepper
Fresh basil leaves, to garnish

- Dry stir-fry the sesame seeds for about a minute then set aside.
- Arrange the vegetables in a single layer, skin uppermost, on a metal grill-tray. Brush with olive oil and place under a medium grill (no closer than 8 cm to the heat) for 7–8 minutes.
- Remove from the grill, and peel the skin from the peppers, onions and tomatoes.
- Season to taste, and sprinkle the lightly toasted sesame seeds over the vegetables.
- Garnish with fresh basil leaves.

Carbohydrate content: 25 grams

Mozzarella aubergine slices with pesto sauce

1 large aubergine, washed and finely sliced lengthways
Sea salt
3 tbsp extra-virgin olive oil
1 medium garlic clove, peeled and finely chopped
2 tbsp coriander pesto sauce (page 225)
75 grams mozzarella cheese, sliced very finely
Freshly ground black pepper
1 tbsp chopped fresh chives, to garnish
Fresh coriander leaves, washed, to garnish

- Place the aubergine slices in a colander, sprinkle with salt and leave for 20–30 minutes. Rinse with cold water and pat dry.
- Heat the olive oil in a large, shallow frying pan then lightly fry the aubergine slices and garlic for 2–3 minutes, turning once.
- Spoon the pesto sauce evenly on each of the aubergine slices, top with the finely sliced mozzarella and place under a hot grill (no closer than 8–10 cm to the heat) for 3–4 minutes, or until the mozzarella just begins to 'bubble'.
- Serve the mozzarella aubergine slices on warmed plates, season to taste and garnish with chopped fresh chives and coriander leaves.

Carbohydrate content per serving: 6 grams

Aubergine kebabs (FOR 2)

1 medium aubergine, chopped into medium chunks
6 plum tomatoes, halved
1 medium red pepper, deseeded and chopped into chunks
1 medium yellow pepper, deseeded and chopped into
    chunks
6 button mushrooms, halved
Rocket and olive salad (page 147)
Lime wedges, to garnish

Marinade
1 tbsp extra-virgin olive oil
1 tbsp chopped fresh basil leaves
1 tbsp chopped fresh parsley
2 tbsp freshly squeezed lime juice
1 garlic clove, peeled and finely chopped

- Mix together the marinade ingredients in a medium mixing bowl.
- Stir in the vegetables.
- Set aside to chill in the fridge for at least 45 minutes.
- Meanwhile, soak some wooden skewers in water.
- Thread the vegetables on to the wooden skewers, alternating the vegetables.
- Place under a medium grill (no closer than 8–10 cm to the heat) for about 8–10 minutes.
- Serve immediately with rocket and olive salad, garnished with lime wedges.

Carbohydrate content per serving: 11 grams

Spinach with chilli and pine nuts (FOR 2)

200 grams spinach
2 tbsp pine nuts
2 tbsp extra-virgin olive oil
2 spring onions, chopped into 3–4 cm lengths
1 garlic clove, peeled and chopped finely
1 small red chilli, deseeded and chopped finely (optional)
Pinch of rock salt
Freshly ground black pepper
Lemon vinaigrette (page 222)

- Lightly steam the spinach for 3–4 minutes, and set aside.
- Meanwhile, lightly toast the pine nuts in a dry pan, and set aside.
- Heat the olive oil in a small frying pan and gently sauté the spring onions, garlic and chilli (if using) for 3–4 minutes.
- Mix together the spinach, pine nuts, spring onions, garlic and chilli, and season to taste.
- Drizzle over lemon vinaigrette.

Carbohydrate content per serving: 3 grams

Baked peppers with mozzarella (FOR 4)

2 tbsp extra-virgin olive oil
2 medium onions, peeled and chopped finely
2 garlic cloves, peeled and chopped finely
2 tsp tomato purée
4 large vine-ripened tomatoes, peeled and diced
1 tbsp chopped fresh oregano
Freshly ground black pepper
4 large yellow peppers, tops removed and deseeded
2 slices of prosciutto ham, diced
4 thick slices of mozzarella cheese
Fresh basil leaves, to garnish

- Preheat the oven to 140°C (gas mark 1).
- Heat the olive oil in a saucepan and lightly sauté the onions and garlic for 1–2 minutes.
- Stir in the tomato purée.
- Pour the mixture into a bowl and add the diced tomatoes and oregano.
- Season to taste and mix thoroughly.
- Spoon the mixture into the peppers, and place the peppers on a baking tray, adding a little water to the tray.
- Cook in the centre of the oven for 30–35 minutes.
- Remove from the oven, sprinkle over the prosciutto ham, top with slices of mozzarella cheese and place under a medium grill for 1–2 minutes, until the cheese has melted.
- Serve immediately, garnished with fresh basil leaves.

Carbohydrate content per serving: 10 grams

Pepperonata

3 tbsp extra-virgin olive oil
1 large red onion, peeled and chopped
1 garlic clove, peeled and chopped finely
4 medium red peppers, deseeded and sliced finely
400-gram tin of plum tomatoes
1 tbsp chopped fresh basil (or 1 tsp dried basil)
1 tbsp chopped fresh parsley (optional)
Freshly ground black pepper

- Heat the olive oil in a medium frying pan and sauté the onion and garlic for 1–2 minutes.
- Stir in the peppers and stir-fry for a further 3–4 minutes.
- Drain the tomatoes.
- Add the tomatoes, basil and parsley (if using), and simmer gently over a low heat for 3–4 minutes.
- Season to taste and serve immediately.

Carbohydrate content per serving: 10 grams

Ratatouille   (FOR 2)

1 medium aubergine, cubed
Pinch of rock salt
3 tbsp extra-virgin olive oil
2 courgettes, chopped
1 medium red pepper, deseeded and chopped
1 medium yellow pepper, deseeded and chopped
1 large onion, peeled and sliced
1 garlic clove, peeled and chopped finely
3 large plum tomatoes, peeled and chopped
75 ml tomato juice
1 tbsp tomato purée
Pinch of granulated sugar
1 bay leaf
1 tbsp chopped fresh basil
1 tsp chopped fresh oregano
Freshly ground black pepper
Fresh basil leaves, to garnish

- Place the chopped aubergine into a colander, sprinkle with salt and allow to stand for 20–30 minutes. Rinse with cold water and pat dry.
- Heat 2 tbsp extra-virgin olive oil in a large frying pan (or preferably a wok) until hot, add the aubergine, courgettes and peppers, and sauté for 2 minutes. Remove with a perforated spoon and cover.
- Heat the remaining olive oil in the pan and sauté the onion and garlic. Add the tomatoes, tomato juice, purée, sugar and bay leaf, and cook for 5–6 minutes.
- Return the aubergine, courgettes and peppers to the pan, and stir in the basil and oregano.

- Season to taste and simmer for a further 2 minutes. Remove the bay leaf and serve, garnished with fresh basil leaves.

Carbohydrate content per serve: 16 grams

Herb tomatoes (FOR 2)

1 garlic clove, peeled and chopped finely
25 grams chopped fresh basil
25 grams chopped fresh flat-leaf parsley
2 beefsteak tomatoes, halved
10 grams fresh breadcrumbs
1 tbsp extra-virgin olive oil
Pinch of rock salt
Freshly ground black pepper
Chopped fresh chives, to garnish

- Preheat the oven to 180°C (gas mark 4).
- Mix together the garlic, basil and parsley.
- Add 3–4 tbsp of water to a shallow casserole dish then place the tomatoes (cut side uppermost) in the dish.
- Divide the garlic and herb mixture between the 4 tomato halves, top with breadcrumbs, drizzle over a little olive oil and season to taste.
- Bake in the centre of the oven for 10–12 minutes.
- Serve immediately, garnished with chopped chives.

Carbohydrate content per serving: 8 grams

Avocado with Bocconcini cheese (FOR 1)

½ medium, ripe Hass avocado, peeled, stone removed and
    diced
50 grams (approximately) Bocconcini cheese, cubed
3 small plum tomatoes on the vine, quartered
2 spring onions, chopped finely
Drizzle of balsamic vinegar
30 grams (approximately) rocket leaves
Freshly ground black pepper

- Mix together the avocado, Bocconcini, tomatoes and
  spring onions in a medium bowl and drizzle over some
  balsamic vinegar.
- Put a bed of rocket leaves on a plate and top with the
  balsamic avocado mixture.
- Season to taste with black pepper.

Carbohydrate content per serving: 4 grams

Traditional cauliflower cheese (FOR 2)

½ a medium cauliflower, washed and chopped into florets
Pinch of rock salt
Freshly ground black pepper
15 grams Parmesan cheese, grated
1 tbsp chopped, fresh flat-leaf parsley

Cheese sauce
25 grams butter
25 grams wholemeal flour
150 ml full-cream milk
30 grams Cheddar cheese, grated

- Place the cauliflower florets in a medium saucepan and add water until just covered.
- Add a pinch of rock salt, bring to the boil and simmer for 8–10 minutes.

At the same time:

- Melt the butter in a medium saucepan, then remove from the heat and stir in the flour to form a smooth roux.
- Return to a gentle heat and gradually add the milk, stirring constantly.
- When the sauce begins to thicken, remove from the heat and stir in the Cheddar cheese.
- Return to the heat, stirring constantly, until the cheese has completely melted.

continued overleaf

- Place the cauliflower florets in a heatproof dish and pour over the cheese sauce.
- Season to taste with black pepper, sprinkle over the Parmesan cheese and place under a hot grill (no closer than 8–10 cm to the heat) for 1–2 minutes until the Parmesan begins to brown.
- Sprinkle over the flat-leaf parsley and serve immediately.

Carbohydrate content per serving: 16 grams

Steamed courgettes with garlic   (FOR 2)

150 grams courgettes, chopped diagonally into 2 cm
   chunks
25 grams unsalted butter
1 medium garlic clove, peeled and finely chopped
50 grams button mushrooms, wiped and halved
Freshly ground black pepper

- Lightly steam the courgettes for 5 minutes (or microwave on 'high' for 2–3 minutes).
- Melt the butter in a medium saucepan and sauté the garlic and mushrooms for 1–2 minutes.
- Put the courgettes on a serving plate and top with the mushrooms and garlic.
- Season to taste with black pepper and serve immediately.

Carbohydrate content per serving: 3 grams

Vegetable stir-fry with pumpkin seeds (FOR 2)

2 tbsp extra-virgin olive oil
100 grams French beans, chopped diagonally into 3 cm
    lengths
100 grams small broccoli florets
1 small red pepper, deseeded and finely sliced
1 medium yellow pepper, deseeded and finely sliced
4 spring onions, chopped
2 slices of fresh root ginger, peeled and finely chopped
1 medium garlic clove, peeled and finely chopped
50 grams baby spinach leaves
1 tbsp soy sauce
1 tbsp dry sherry
Freshly ground black pepper
1 tbsp pumpkin seeds

- Heat the olive oil in a wok and stir-fry the French beans, broccoli, peppers, spring onions, ginger, garlic and spinach leaves for 4–5 minutes.
- Stir in the soy sauce and sherry and cook for a further 2 minutes.
- Season to taste and serve immediately, sprinkled with the pumpkin seeds.

Carbohydrate content per serving: 12 grams

Green veggie frittata (FOR 2)

50 grams asparagus, sliced diagonally into 3 cm lengths
50 grams mangetout
50 grams green beans, sliced diagonally into 3 cm lengths
4 medium organic free-range eggs
2 tbsp full-cream milk
25 grams unsalted butter
2 spring onions, peeled and chopped
30 grams freshly grated Parmesan cheese
Freshly ground black pepper
1 tbsp chopped chives
1 tbsp sunflower seeds, to garnish

- Cook the asparagus, mangetout and green beans in boiling water for about 3 minutes (or steam for 4–5 minutes), then drain and set aside.
- Beat the eggs in a medium mixing bowl with the milk.
- Melt the butter in a medium frying pan and pour in the egg mixture.
- Cook gently, stirring occasionally, until the mixture begins to set.
- Remove the pan from the heat and stir in the cooked vegetables, spring onions and Parmesan cheese.
- Return the pan to the heat for 1–2 minutes.
- Serve immediately, seasoned with black pepper and garnished with chopped chives and sunflower seeds.

Carbohydrate content per serving: 6 grams

Savoy cabbage with ginger (FOR 2)

1 tbsp sesame seeds
2 tbsp extra-virgin olive oil
4 slices fresh root ginger, peeled and sliced
1 small red chilli, deseeded and finely chopped
3 spring onions, chopped into 3 cm lengths
½ Savoy cabbage, finely shredded
1 tsp sesame oil

- Place the sesame seeds in a small frying pan and dry-cook for 1–2 minutes. Set aside.
- Heat the oil in a wok and stir-fry the ginger, chilli, spring onions and cabbage for 4–5 minutes.
- Stir in the sesame seeds and drizzle over a few drops of sesame oil.
- Serve immediately.

Carbohydrate content per serving: 4 grams

Semi-dried tomatoes with herbs   (FOR 4)

8 large plum tomatoes, quartered lengthways
1 tbsp chopped fresh basil
1 tbsp chopped fresh thyme
Freshly ground black pepper
2 tbsp extra-virgin olive oil

- Place the tomatoes skin down on a wire rack in a baking tray, sprinkle with the herbs and pepper and cook in the centre of a pre-heated oven at 150°C (gas mark 2) for about 2½–3 hours.
- Remove from the oven, mix with extra-virgin olive oil and cool in the fridge for 3–4 hours before use.

Carbohydrate content per serving: 6 grams

Baby leeks in lemon butter sauce (FOR 2)

6 baby leeks
50 grams unsalted butter
3 tbsp freshly squeezed lemon juice

■ Place the baby leeks in a microwave-safe container, add 2 tbsp water, cover and microwave on 'high' for 3 minutes.

Or

■ Lightly steam the baby leeks for about 10 minutes.

At the same time:

■ Melt the butter in a small saucepan, stir in the lemon juice and heat through gently for about a minute.
■ Serve the leeks and pour over the lemon butter sauce.

Carbohydrate content per serving: 2 grams

Chapter 16 Dressings and Sauces

Mayonnaise

2 egg yolks from large, free-range eggs
1 garlic clove, peeled and finely chopped
1 tsp Dijon mustard
1 tsp white wine vinegar
200 ml extra-virgin olive oil
Pinch of rock salt
Freshly ground black pepper

- Place the egg yolks, garlic, mustard and white wine vinegar in a food processor and blend for a few seconds, then – with the motor running – add the olive oil slowly and evenly.
- Season to taste, adding a little extra white wine vinegar if necessary.

Carbohydrate content per serving: negligible

Mustard vinaigrette

4 tbsp extra-virgin olive oil
1 tbsp white wine vinegar
1 tbsp wholegrain mustard
1 small garlic clove, peeled and grated

■ Add the ingredients of the vinaigrette to a large screw-top jar and shake vigorously to mix.

Carbohydrate content per serve: 1 gram

French vinaigrette (FOR 8)

250 ml extra-virgin olive oil
75 ml white wine vinegar
2 tsp dry mustard powder
1 large garlic clove, peeled and grated
Freshly ground black pepper

■ Add the ingredients of the vinaigrette to a large screw-top jar and shake vigorously to mix.

Carbohydrate content per serving: <1 gram

Balsamic vinaigrette (FOR 8)

250 ml extra-virgin olive oil
75 ml balsamic vinegar
1 large garlic clove, peeled and grated
Freshly ground black pepper

- Add the ingredients of the vinaigrette to a large screw-top jar and shake vigorously to mix.

Carbohydrate content per serving: 2 grams

Lemon vinaigrette (FOR 8)

250 ml extra-virgin olive oil
75 ml white wine vinegar
60 ml freshly squeezed lemon juice
Freshly ground black pepper

- Add the ingredients of the vinaigrette to a large screw-top jar and shake vigorously to mix.

Carbohydrate content per serving: <1 gram

Oriental vinaigrette (FOR 2)

5 tbsp extra-virgin olive oil
1 tbsp white wine vinegar
1 tbsp light soy sauce
1 tbsp sweet sherry
1 tsp sesame oil
1 slice of fresh ginger root, peeled and finely chopped
Freshly ground black pepper

- Add the ingredients of the vinaigrette to a large screw-top jar and shake vigorously to mix.

Carbohydrate content per serving: 1 gram

Passata vinaigrette

3 tbsp extra-virgin olive oil
3 tbsp passata (or tomato juice)
1 tbsp red wine vinegar
½ garlic clove, peeled and grated
Pinch of rock salt
Freshly ground black pepper

- Add the ingredients of the vinaigrette to a large screw-top jar and shake vigorously to mix.

Carbohydrate content per serving: 3 grams

Tomato sauce

400-gram tin of peeled plum tomatoes
1 tbsp tomato purée
1 tsp granulated sugar
1 tbsp chopped fresh basil or 1 tsp dried basil (optional)
Freshly ground black pepper
Dash of Worcester sauce

- Drain the tomatoes, reserving the juice, and pour into a small saucepan.
- Stir in the tomato purée, sugar and herbs (if using), and season to taste with black pepper.
- Add 1 tbsp of tomato juice to the pan and bring to a gentle simmer for 5 minutes.
- Add a dash of Worcester sauce to the remaining tomato juice and enjoy!

Carbohydrate content per serving: 6 grams

Cucumber raita

200 ml natural yoghurt
1 tbsp chopped fresh mint
½ tsp ground cumin
1 small Lebanese cucumber, diced

- Mix together the yoghurt, mint, cumin and cucumber in a small bowl, cover and cool in the fridge.

Carbohydrate content per serving: 2 grams

Coriander pesto sauce (FOR 2)

30 grams fresh coriander leaves
1 garlic clove, peeled and chopped
25 grams pine nuts
25 grams grated Parmesan cheese
Pinch of rock salt
Freshly ground black pepper
40 ml extra-virgin olive oil

- Add the coriander, garlic, pine nuts, cheese and seasoning to a blender and blend until finely chopped.
- Gradually add the olive oil while blending.

Carbohydrate content per serving: 1 gram

Basil pesto sauce (FOR 8)

100 grams pine nuts
150 grams chopped fresh basil leaves
2 garlic cloves, peeled
100 grams Parmesan cheese, grated
Freshly ground black pepper
150 ml extra-virgin olive oil

- Dry stir-fry the pine nuts for 1–2 minutes.
- Blend the pine nuts, basil, garlic, Parmesan cheese and pepper in a blender or food processor.
- Gradually add the extra-virgin olive oil while blending.

Carbohydrate content per serving: 2 grams

Rocket and mint sauce   (FOR 2)

75 ml sour cream
1 tbsp chopped fresh wild rocket leaves
1 tbsp chopped fresh mint leaves
Pinch of cayenne pepper

■   Mix together the sour cream, chopped rocket and
    mint leaves and cayenne pepper in a medium bowl.
■   Cover and cool in the fridge for 20–30 minutes before
    use.

Carbohydrate content per serving: 2 grams

Mango raita   (FOR 2)

100 ml natural yoghurt
¼ medium cucumber, peeled and diced
2 tsp chopped fresh coriander
¼ ripe mango, diced
Fresh mint leaves, to garnish

■   Blend together the yoghurt, cucumber, coriander and
    mango then set aside to cool in the fridge for at least
    20 minutes.
■   Garnish with fresh mint leaves and serve immediately.

Carbohydrate content per serving: 11 grams

Chapter 17 The Maintenance Phase

The maintenance phase of the Diabetes Revolution is the same for both type 1 and type 2 diabetics. By this time the diabetes will be better controlled with either a reduced need for insulin injections (in type 1 diabetics) or simply lower levels of serum insulin and therefore lower blood sugar levels with less medication in type 2 diabetics. You can now reintroduce many of the foods that were excluded during the initial phase of the programme. These include whole grains, wholegrain rice, wholemeal pasta, fruit, pulses and desserts.

You can include any of these foods, **but in moderation**.

It is important to remember that if you feast exclusively on high-GI/high-carbohydrate foods, then diabetic control will be lost once again.

Introduce the higher-GI meals in moderation, checking blood sugars on a daily basis while you amend your diet. It isn't essential to measure blood sugars as regularly when you achieve stability, but in the initial stages of changing the dietary programme this is essential.

Initially, we suggest you introduce one food group only each week. In the first week you may wish to introduce two pasta dishes; in the second week perhaps increase fruit intake to two pieces per day, and so on. We wouldn't advise having more than three high-GI/high-carb meals per week, and certainly no more than four pieces of fruit per day. If you add too many of the high-GI/high-carb foods into the diet this will significantly impair glucose tolerance and control of blood sugars.

When blood sugar levels begin to rise, or your requirement for insulin (by injection) increases, this is a warning that your intake of high-GI foods is too high and should be reduced.

Snacks

Snacks shouldn't really be necessary in a well-balanced diet. If you eat three or four substantial meals that raise blood sugar slowly each day, your energy levels should be sustained. However, no system is perfect so we have to allow for times when you might need some extra energy, particularly in the early stages of the programme when blood sugars will not be entirely controlled. Snacks that are particularly useful in this regard include:

- nuts (except pistachios, cashew nuts, peanuts and chestnuts)
- an extra piece of fruit (not banana or mango) or a bowl of berries such as blueberries, blackberries, raspberries or strawberries
- yoghurt (low-sugar and low-fat)
- fresh vegetables crudités such as celery, cucumber and carrots

- melon (four slices of honeydew or rock melon)
- seeds such as linseed, flaxseed or sunflower seeds

Main Courses

Penne rigate with mixed veggies (FOR 2)

25 grams mangetout
25 grams broccoli florets
1 small red pepper, deseeded and finely sliced
40 grams wholemeal penne rigate
75 ml crème fraîche
1 tbsp freshly chopped basil
1 tbsp freshly grated Parmesan cheese
Freshly ground black pepper

- Lightly steam the mangetout, broccoli florets and red pepper for 4–5 minutes (or microwave on 'high' for 2–3 minutes).

At the same time:

- Cook the penne rigate according to packet instructions, and drain.
- Mix together the crème fraîche and basil.
- Add the mangetout, broccoli and red peppers to the penne rigate, stir in the crème fraîche and Parmesan cheese and season to taste with black pepper.

Carbohydrate content per serving: 20 grams

Fettucine with chicken and basil (FOR 2)

2 medium chicken breasts (about 150 grams each)
25 grams butter, cubed
60 grams fettucine
2 tbsp extra-virgin olive oil
1 medium brown onion, peeled and chopped
50 grams button mushrooms, wiped and sliced
2 tbsp sun-dried tomatoes in extra-virgin olive oil, drained
     and finely sliced
1 tbsp chopped fresh basil leaves
4 green olives, finely sliced
1 tbsp freshly grated Parmesan cheese
Freshly ground black pepper

Sauce
15 grams unsalted butter
2 tsp plain wholemeal flour
75 ml full-cream milk

- Preheat the oven to 180°C (gas mark 4).
- Place the chicken breasts in an ovenproof dish, dot with butter cubes, cover with pierced aluminium foil and cook in the centre of the oven for 35–40 minutes.
- Remove from the oven and set aside to cool then slice finely.

Just before the chicken has cooked:

- Put the dried pasta into a large pan of boiling water and cook for about 8 minutes (or 3–4 minutes for fresh pasta). Drain.

- Heat the olive oil in a medium frying pan and sauté the onion and mushrooms for 3–4 minutes.
- Prepare the sauce. Melt the butter in a medium saucepan, remove from the heat and stir in the flour to form a smooth roux.
- Return to the heat and add the milk, stirring constantly.
- As the sauce thickens, remove from the heat.
- Add the chicken, onion, mushrooms, sun-dried tomatoes and basil to the fettucine in a large bowl then gently stir in the sauce.
- Serve immediately, garnished with olives and Parmesan cheese.
- Season to taste.

Carbohydrate content per serving: 30 grams

Pecorino fettucine with herbs　(FOR 2)

2 tbsp extra-virgin olive oil
3 shallots, peeled and diced
2 medium garlic cloves, peeled and finely chopped
60 grams fettucine
1 tbsp unsalted butter
100 grams chopped fresh spinach leaves
1 tbsp chopped fresh sage (or basil)
1 tbsp freshly grated Pecorino cheese
Freshly ground black pepper

- Heat the olive oil in a small frying pan and sauté the shallots and garlic for 1–2 minutes.

At the same time:

- Cook the fettucine until *al dente*.
- Melt the butter in a medium saucepan and cook the spinach and sage (or basil) for 30–60 seconds until it just begins to soften, then remove from the heat immediately.
- Stir the shallots, garlic, spinach, sage and Pecorino cheese into the fettucine, season with black pepper and serve immediately.

Carbohydrate content per serving: 25 grams

Tagliatelli carbonara (FOR 2)

40 grams dried wholemeal tagliatelli
1 fresh salmon steak (approximately 125–150 grams)
Extra-virgin olive oil
100 ml double cream
40 grams freshly grated Parmesan cheese
Freshly ground black pepper
1 tbsp freshly chopped flat-leaf parsley

- Cook the tagliatelli according to the packet instructions.

At the same time:

- Brush the salmon steak with olive oil.
- Cook the salmon for 6 minutes under a medium grill (no closer than 10 cm to the heat), turning once.
- Allow the salmon to cool for a few minutes, then flake the salmon steak, removing all bones and skin.
- Whisk the cream until slightly thickened.
- When the tagliatelli is cooked, drain and transfer to a large, warm bowl. Stir in the flaked salmon, cream and grated Parmesan.
- Season to taste then serve immediately, garnished with fresh parsley.

Carbohydrate content per serving: 16 grams

Wholemeal spaghetti Napolitana (FOR 2)

40 grams wholemeal spaghetti

Napolitana sauce
2 tbsp extra-virgin olive oil
4 shallots, peeled and finely chopped
1 medium garlic clove, peeled and finely chopped
50 grams button mushrooms, wiped and sliced
440-gram tin of plum tomatoes
75 ml passata
1 tsp dried oregano
1 tsp dried basil
Pinch of salt
Freshly ground black pepper

- Heat the olive oil in a large frying pan and sauté the shallots and garlic for 2–3 minutes.
- Stir in the mushrooms and sauté for a further minute.
- Stir in the tomatoes, oregano and basil, season to taste and simmer gently for 5–7 minutes.

At the same time:

- Cook the spaghetti according to the packet instructions.
- When the spaghetti is cooked, drain, stir in the Napolitana sauce and serve immediately.

Carbohydrate content per serving: 26 grams

Penne with char-grilled vegetables (FOR 2)

1 medium red onion, peeled and quartered
2 courgettes, chopped diagonally into 2–3 cm chunks
1 medium green pepper, deseeded and quartered
1 medium red pepper, deseeded and quartered
3 cherry tomatoes, halved
2 medium garlic cloves, peeled and finely chopped
2 tbsp extra-virgin olive oil
60 grams penne pasta
2 tbsp freshly grated Parmesan cheese
1 tbsp chopped fresh basil leaves
Freshly ground black pepper
Passata vinaigrette (page 223)

- Place the vegetables on a grill tray, skin uppermost, sprinkling the chopped garlic over them.
- Drizzle with the olive oil and place under a medium grill (no closer than 8–10 cm to the heat) for 5–7 minutes, turning twice.
- Remove from the heat and allow to cool for 1–2 minutes. Peel the skin from the peppers and tomatoes and slice the peppers thinly.

At the same time:

- Cook the penne until *al dente*.
- Serve the vegetables on a bed of penne and top with freshly grated Parmesan and basil.
- Season to taste and serve immediately.

Carbohydrate content per serving: 29 grams

Pappardelle with two   (FOR 2)
cheese sauce

50 grams sun-dried tomatoes
50 grams freshly grated Parmesan cheese
1 tbsp ricotta cheese
1 tbsp chopped fresh coriander leaves
1 tbsp chopped fresh basil leaves
2 tbsp extra-virgin olive oil
60 grams pappardelle
Freshly ground black pepper

- Blend together the tomatoes, Parmesan and ricotta cheese, coriander, basil and olive oil.
- Cook the pappardelle until *al dente*.
- Drain the pappardelle, stir through the sauce and heat gently for 1–2 minutes then season to taste and serve immediately.

Carbohydrate content per serving: 25 grams

Spaghetti Bolognese (FOR 2)

40 grams wholemeal spaghetti

Bolognese sauce
3 tbsp extra-virgin olive oil
1 medium red onion, peeled and chopped
2 garlic cloves, peeled and finely chopped
200 grams turkey mince (or vegetarian mince)
1 tbsp tomato purée
150 ml chicken stock
1 tbsp chopped fresh basil leaves (or 1 tsp dried basil)
Freshly ground black pepper

- Heat the olive oil in a medium frying pan.
- Sauté the onion and garlic for 2–3 minutes.
- Add the turkey mince and stir regularly until browned.
- Stir in the tomato purée, stock and basil, season to taste and simmer gently for 5–7 minutes.

At the same time:

- Cook the spaghetti according to the packet instructions.
- Serve the spaghetti with the Bolognese sauce.

Carbohydrate content per serving: 20 grams

Lasagne   (FOR 4)

Bolognese sauce (see page 237)
30 grams unsalted butter
30 grams plain flour
150 ml milk
4 sheets of dried lasagne
1 tbsp freshly grated Parmesan cheese
100 grams fresh watercress
2 tbsp balsamic vinegar
Freshly ground black pepper

- Prepare the Bolognese sauce.
- Preheat the oven to 180°C (gas mark 4).
- Melt the butter in a medium saucepan then remove from the heat and stir in the flour until the mixture is smooth.
- Return the pan to a gentle heat and gradually add the milk, stirring constantly, until the sauce just begins to thicken. Remove from the heat, continuing to stir.
- Spread about a quarter of the Bolognese sauce over the base of a loaf tin, top with white sauce then cover with a sheet of lasagne.
- Repeat this 3 times then cover the final sheet of lasagne with the remaining white sauce, sprinkle over the grated Parmesan cheese and cook in the centre of the oven for 30 minutes.
- Divide the lasagne into 4 equal portions and serve immediately with fresh watercress.
- Drizzle a little balsamic vinegar over the watercress and season to taste.

Carbohydrate content per serving: 20 grams

Classic macaroni cheese (FOR 2)

30 grams unsalted butter
30 grams wholemeal flour
½ tsp dry mustard
150 ml full-cream milk
40 grams Cheddar cheese, grated
1 tbsp chopped fresh basil leaves
1 tbsp chopped fresh flat-leaf parsley
Freshly ground black pepper
50 grams organic macaroni
100 grams fresh rocket leaves

- Melt the butter in a medium saucepan and stir in the flour and dry mustard.
- Remove from the heat and gradually add the milk, stirring constantly.
- Return to a moderate heat, continuing to stir, until the mixture just begins to thicken.
- Stir in the cheese, basil leaves and flat-leaf parsley, and season to taste.

At the same time:

- Cook the macaroni in a large saucepan of boiling water for 8–10 minutes.
- Stir the macaroni into the sauce and serve immediately with fresh rocket.

Carbohydrate content per serving: 34 grams

Angel hair pasta with Italian sauce   (FOR 2)

60 grams angel hair pasta
1 tbsp chopped fresh flat-leaf parsley
Freshly ground black pepper

Italian sauce
1 tbsp extra-virgin olive oil
1 medium shallot, peeled and finely chopped
1 garlic clove, peeled and finely chopped
2 slices fresh root ginger, peeled and finely chopped
50 grams button mushrooms, wiped and sliced
100 ml dry white wine
1 tbsp freshly squeezed lime juice
1 tsp tomato purée
1 tsp dried oregano

- Heat the olive oil in a medium frying pan and sauté the shallot, garlic, ginger and mushrooms for 2 minutes.
- Add the dry white wine, lime juice, tomato purée and oregano, and simmer gently for 2–3 minutes.

At the same time:

- Cook the angel hair pasta in a large pan of boiling water for 2 minutes.
- Toss the pasta with the sauce, stir in the parsley and season to taste.

Carbohydrate content per serving: 27 grams

Milanese risotto (FOR 2)

2 tbsp extra-virgin olive oil
1 small red onion, peeled and finely chopped
1 medium garlic clove, peeled and finely chopped
1 medium red pepper, deseeded and chopped
1 medium yellow pepper, deseeded and chopped
2 slices fresh root ginger, peeled and finely chopped
60 grams arborio rice
3 tbsp dry white wine
200 ml chicken (or vegetable) stock
½ tsp saffron powder
1 tbsp freshly grated Parmesan cheese
1 tbsp chopped fresh parsley
Freshly ground black pepper

- Heat the olive oil in a medium frying pan and sauté the onion, garlic and peppers for 1–2 minutes.
- Stir in the ginger and rice and cook for 1 minute.
- Add the wine and simmer gently for 1 minute.
- Stir in the stock and saffron powder and simmer gently until the rice is cooked and most of the liquid is absorbed.
- Stir in the Parmesan cheese and cook for a further minute then remove from the heat, top with fresh parsley, season to taste with black pepper and serve immediately.

Carbohydrate content per serving: 30 grams

Button mushroom and basil risotto   (FOR 2)

2 tbsp groundnut oil
1 small onion, peeled and finely chopped
1 medium garlic clove, peeled and finely chopped
100 grams button mushrooms, wiped and halved
60 grams arborio rice
200 ml chicken (or vegetable) stock
1 tbsp chopped fresh basil leaves
1 tbsp chopped fresh mint leaves
Freshly ground black pepper

- Heat the groundnut oil in a medium frying pan then sauté the onion and garlic for 1–2 minutes.
- Add the mushrooms and stir-fry for 3–4 minutes.
- Stir in the rice and add the stock.
- Simmer over a gentle heat for 8–10 minutes, stirring frequently, then stir in the basil and mint leaves.
- Simmer gently for a further 6–8 minutes until the rice is cooked then season to taste with black pepper and serve immediately.

Carbohydrate content per serving: 26 grams

Chilli con carne (FOR 2)

2 tbsp extra-virgin olive oil
1 medium red onion, peeled and chopped
2 medium garlic cloves, peeled and chopped
200 grams turkey mince (or vegetarian mince)
1 level tbsp wholemeal flour
½ tsp chilli powder (optional)
1 tbsp tomato purée
200 ml chicken stock (or Swiss bouillon vegetable stock)
50 grams tinned red kidney beans, drained
50 grams wholegrain rice

- Heat the olive oil in a medium frying pan and sauté the onion and garlic for 1–2 minutes.
- Add the mince and brown.
- Stir in the flour, chilli powder (if using) and tomato purée, then gradually add the stock.
- Add the kidney beans and simmer gently for 10 minutes.

At the same time:

- Cook the rice.
- Serve the chilli mince with the rice.

Carbohydrate content per serving: 31 grams

Smoked haddock kedgeree   (FOR 2)

2 medium smoked haddock fillets (approximately
    150 grams each)
25 grams unsalted butter, cubed
50 grams wholegrain rice
2 tbsp extra-virgin olive oil
1 medium red onion, peeled and chopped
½ tsp medium curry powder
1 large free-range hard-boiled egg, peeled and chopped
1 tbsp each chopped fresh basil and parsley
Freshly ground black pepper

- Preheat the oven to 180°C (gas mark 4).
- Place the haddock fillets in a medium, ovenproof baking dish, dot with butter and cover with pierced aluminium foil.
- Cook in the centre of the oven for 20 minutes, then remove from the heat and flake the haddock.

At the same time:

- Cook the rice.
- Heat the olive oil in a medium frying pan and sauté the onion for 1–2 minutes.
- Stir in the curry powder and cook for a few seconds, then stir in the cooked rice, egg, flaked haddock, basil and parsley.
- Cook over a gentle heat for 2–3 minutes then season to taste and serve immediately.

Carbohydrate content per serving: 20 grams

Chow mein

60 grams Chinese egg noodles
1 tsp rock salt
150 grams peeled, cooked prawns (or tofu)
2 tbsp groundnut oil
100 grams bamboo shoots
75 grams mangetout (or Chinese cabbage, shredded)
2 slices of fresh root ginger, peeled and finely chopped
75 grams bean sprouts
Few drops of sesame oil
Freshly ground black pepper
1 spring onion, finely chopped, to garnish

Marinade
2 tbsp light soy sauce
1 tbsp rice wine or dry sherry
½ tsp cornflour
½ tsp caster sugar
1 tsp grated fresh root ginger

- Add the Chinese egg noodles to 1.5 litres of water in a large saucepan, stir in a tsp of rock salt and bring to the boil.
- Cook for 3–4 minutes then drain.

At the same time:

- Combine the marinade ingredients and marinate the prawns for 30–60 minutes.

continued overleaf

- Heat the groundnut oil in a wok and stir-fry the bamboo shoots, mangetout and ginger for 1–2 minutes.
- Stir in the marinated prawns and bean sprouts then stir-fry for another 2 minutes.
- Stir in the noodles, heat through for a further minute then season to taste with sesame oil and black pepper and serve immediately, garnished with finely chopped spring onion.

Carbohydrate content per serving: 30 grams

Vegetable quiche   (FOR 4)

Pastry

100 grams plain wholemeal flour
50 grams butter
Cold water

Vegetable filling

25 grams asparagus tips
25 grams small broccoli florets
1 small leek, peeled and chopped
1 medium courgette, shaved finely
1 medium tomato on the vine, sliced thinly
30 grams Parmesan cheese, freshly grated
1 tbsp chopped fresh basil
2 medium organic free-range eggs
100 ml full-cream milk
Freshly ground black pepper
Green salad (page 139)

- Add the flour to a medium mixing bowl then rub in the butter.
- Add a little cold water to form a stiff dough.
- Lightly grease a medium (15 cm) flan tin with butter.
- Roll the dough reasonably thinly, line the flan tin and chill in the fridge for 15 minutes.
- Preheat the oven to 180°C (gas mark 4).
- Place baking paper over the pastry case and weight down with baking beads.
- Put the tin in the oven for about 10 minutes, then reduce the temperature to 170°C (gas mark 3) for 2–3 minutes.
- Remove from the oven and set aside to cool.
- Bring a medium saucepan of water to the boil, add the asparagus, broccoli, leek and courgette and cook for 2–3 minutes.
- Drain the vegetables and transfer them to the pastry case.
- Top with slices of tomato and sprinkle over the Parmesan cheese and chopped basil leaves.
- Beat the eggs and milk together and pour into the flan case.
- Transfer the flan to a medium oven – 170°C (gas mark 3) – for about 45–50 minutes.
- Season with black pepper and serve immediately with a green salad or allow to chill.

Carbohydrate content per serving: 21 grams

Desserts

Desserts are definitely a no-go area in the early stages of diabetic control. However, you can incorporate them into your diet later without disturbing the delicate balance of diabetes. Here are some delicious recipes which can be included in the maintenance phase.

Dark chocolate mousse (FOR 2)

45 grams dark chocolate (minimum 70 per cent cocoa content)
20 ml fresh full-cream milk
50 ml fresh double cream

- Grate about 5 grams (very little) of the chocolate and set aside.
- Break up the rest of the chocolate into small pieces, place in a heatproof bowl and melt over a pan of gently simmering hot water. Stir the chocolate from the edges of the bowl as it gradually melts.
- Boil the milk then stir it into the chocolate.
- Set aside to cool.
- Whip the double cream until stiff then fold 40 ml of cream into the chocolate.
- Transfer the chocolate mousse to ramekin dishes and top with the remaining cream.
- Sprinkle over the grated chocolate and serve immediately.

Carbohydrate content per serving: 10 grams

Creamy vanilla (white) chocolate mousse   (FOR 2)

Follow the instructions for dark chocolate mousse (opposite), substituting dark chocolate with vanilla chocolate.

Carbohydrate content per serving: 15 grams

Lemon syllabub   (FOR 2)

75 ml dry white wine
1 tbsp freshly squeezed lemon juice
1 tsp finely grated lemon rind
1 tbsp caster sugar
150 ml double cream
Fresh mint leaves, to garnish

- Mix together the white wine, lemon juice, lemon rind and sugar in a medium bowl.
- Stir in the cream and spoon into wine glasses.
- Chill in the fridge for 2–3 hours and serve, garnished with fresh mint leaves.

Carbohydrate content per serving: 13 grams

Orange syllabub   (FOR 2)

1 tbsp caster sugar
4 tbsp freshly squeezed orange juice
100 ml fresh double cream
Pinch of ground nutmeg

- Mix together the caster sugar and orange juice in a medium bowl and stir in the cream.
- Spoon the mixture into tall glasses and chill in the fridge for 2–4 hours. Sprinkle over a pinch of ground nutmeg and serve chilled.

Carbohydrate content per serving: 17 grams

Strawberries with blueberry purée   (FOR 2)

150 grams blueberries, washed
2 tbsp water
25 grams icing sugar
100 ml double cream
200 grams strawberries, washed and hulled

- Place the blueberries, water and sugar in a medium saucepan and simmer for 4–5 minutes.
- Set aside to cool.
- Purée the blueberries. Whip the double cream.
- Place the strawberries on dessert plates, top with whipped cream and serve with the blueberries.

Carbohydrate content per serving: 30 grams

Strawberry cream (FOR 2)

1 tbsp caster sugar
4 tbsp cold water
200 grams fresh strawberries, hulled and sliced
200 ml double cream, whipped

- Dissolve the sugar in the water in a small saucepan.
- Bring to the boil and simmer until reduced to about half.
- Add the strawberries (setting aside 2 strawberries for garnishing) and gently simmer for 5 minutes.
- Blend the mixture and set aside to cool.
- Fold the strawberry purée into the cream.
- Spoon the mixture into dessert dishes and garnish with strawberry slices.

Carbohydrate content per serving: 17 grams

Raspberry cream (FOR 2)

Follow the recipe for strawberry cream (above), substituting raspberries for strawberries.

Carbohydrate content per serving: 16 grams

Strawberries in raspberry cream   (FOR 2)

Raspberry cream (page 251)
100 grams strawberries, washed, hulled and halved
  lengthways

- Prepare the raspberry cream.
- Stir in the strawberries and serve immediately.

Carbohydrate content per serving: 19 grams

Strawberries with orange cream   (FOR 2)

200 grams fresh strawberries, washed and hulled
6 tbsp freshly squeezed orange juice
200 ml double cream
Fresh mint leaves, to garnish

- Mix together the strawberries and orange juice, cover
  and chill in the fridge for 2 hours.
- Transfer the mixture to dessert dishes and top with
  cream.
- Garnish with fresh mint leaves and serve immediately.

Carbohydrate content per serving: 18 grams

Ricotta with soft berries

100 grams blackberries, washed
75 grams ricotta cheese, sliced
2 tsp runny honey
100 grams strawberries, washed, hulled and quartered
    lengthways
Fresh mint leaves, to garnish (optional)

- Purée the blackberries in a blender.
- Arrange the slices of ricotta cheese in the centre of
  the plates and drizzle over the honey.
- Spoon the blackberry purée over the cheese.
- Top with strawberries and mint leaves, if using.

Carbohydrate content per serving: 14 grams

Caramelised berry pudding (FOR 4)

100 ml double cream
100 ml natural yoghurt
150 grams fresh raspberries, washed
150 grams fresh blackberries (or blueberries), washed
25 grams demerara sugar
Fresh mint leaves, to garnish

- Mix together the double cream and yoghurt.
- Place the berries in the base of a heatproof shallow dish.
- Spread the cream and yoghurt mixture over the fruit and chill in the fridge for 1–2 hours.
- Sprinkle the sugar over the cream mixture and place under a medium grill, no closer than 8–10 cm to the heat, until the sugar caramelises.
- Serve immediately, garnished with fresh mint leaves.

Carbohydrate content per serving: 16 grams

Berry fruit fool

150 grams mixed red berries, such as raspberries,
redcurrants and strawberries
4 tbsp water
25 grams caster sugar
1 tbsp freshly squeezed lemon juice
150 ml fresh double cream
4 fresh mint leaves, to garnish

- Place the mixed berries, water, sugar and lemon juice in a medium saucepan, bring to the boil then lower the heat and simmer gently until the fruit softens.
- Blend until smooth and set aside to cool.
- Whisk the cream until firm and fold into the cooled purée.
- Transfer to a medium bowl and chill before serving, garnished with fresh mint leaves.

Carbohydrate content per serving: 18 grams

Custard fruit fool

Follow the recipe for berry fruit fool, above, substituting the cream with baked egg custard (overleaf).

Carbohydrate content per serving: 28 grams

Yoghurt fruit fool

Follow the recipe for berry fruit fool, above, substituting the cream with Greek yoghurt.

Carbohydrate content per serving: 23 grams

Baked egg custard

3 large free-range eggs
500 ml full-cream milk
1½ tbsp caster sugar
Freshly ground nutmeg

- Preheat the oven to 170°C (gas mark 3).
- Beat together the eggs and milk.
- Strain the mixture through a sieve and stir in the caster sugar.
- Pour the mixture into a greased ovenproof dish and sprinkle with freshly ground nutmeg.
- Place the dish in a roasting tin. Pour hot water into the roasting tin to about half the depth of the tin.
- Bake in the centre of the oven for 50–60 minutes.

Carbohydrate content per serving: 13 grams

Crème brûlée

2 large free-range eggs
150 ml double cream
1 tbsp icing sugar
½ tsp vanilla essence
1 tbsp caster sugar

- Separate the yolks from the egg whites and beat the yolks in a medium bowl.
- Pour the cream into a small saucepan and heat gently.
- Remove from the heat then beat the warm cream into the yolk mixture.
- Stir in the icing sugar and vanilla essence.
- Return the mixture to the saucepan and heat very gently (but do not allow to boil), stirring constantly until the mixture thickens.
- Pour into a 500 ml shallow, greased, heatproof dish, and chill in the fridge for at least 4 hours (preferably overnight).
- Just before serving, sprinkle the caster sugar over the mixture, then place under a medium grill, no closer than 8–10 cm to the heat, until the sugar caramelises.
- Remove from the heat and allow to cool before serving.

Carbohydrate content per serving: 18 grams

Crème caramel (FOR 2)

75 ml water
2½ tbsp caster sugar
2 large free-range eggs
¼ tsp vanilla essence
250 ml full-cream milk
75 ml fresh single cream, to serve

- Preheat the oven to 150°C (gas mark 2).
- Pour the water into a small saucepan and stir in 2 tbsp of the sugar.
- Cook over a low heat, stirring constantly, until the sugar has completely dissolved.
- Pour the syrup into 2 ramekins to cover the base.
- Whisk the eggs and stir in the vanilla essence and remaining sugar.
- Pour the milk into a small saucepan and heat gently until warm then remove from the heat.
- Stir the whisked egg mixture into the warm milk.
- Sieve the mixture and pour into the ramekins.
- Place the ramekins in a roasting tin, then pour hot water into the tin to about half the depth of the ramekins.
- Cook in the centre of the oven for 50–60 minutes.
- Remove from the oven and set aside to cool.
- Serve with fresh cream.

Carbohydrate content per serving: 26 grams

Crêpes suzette

6 crêpes (see recipe on page 118)

Sauce
5 tbsp freshly squeezed orange juice
2 tbsp freshly squeezed lemon juice
2 tbsp Cointreau
1 tsp caster sugar
25 grams butter

- Make the crêpes.
- Mix together the orange juice, lemon juice, Cointreau and sugar in a medium mixing bowl.
- Melt the butter in a medium frying pan and gently heat the sauce mixture.
- Lay a crêpe on the citrus mixture in the pan, allow it to absorb the mixture for about 30 seconds then fold the crêpe in half and remove from the pan.
- Do the same for the other crêpes.
- Serve immediately.

Carbohydrate content per serving: 30 grams

Crêpes with apple and cinnamon   FOR 2

Follow the recipe for crêpes suzette, adding ¼ tsp of ground cinnamon and 1 peeled and grated apple.

Carbohydrate content per serving: 26 grams

Crêpes with lemon and cinnamon (FOR 2)

Follow the recipe for crêpes suzette, adding ¼ tsp of ground cinnamon and drizzle 1 tbsp of freshly squeezed lemon juice over each crêpe.

Carbohydrate content per serving: 22 grams

Pears poached in Cabernet Sauvignon (FOR 2)

250 ml Cabernet Sauvignon red wine
25 grams caster sugar
3 cloves
2 large pears, washed and peeled
Sprigs of fresh mint, to garnish

- Pour the wine into a medium saucepan and stir in the sugar and cloves.
- Heat the wine, stirring constantly, until the sugar dissolves.
- Add the pears and simmer gently for 30 minutes, turning the pears occasionally.
- Remove the cloves then serve the pears with the reduced red wine sauce, garnished with sprigs of fresh mint.

Carbohydrate content per serving: 30 grams

Peach and blackberry surprise (FOR 2)

150 grams ripe blackberries
2 ripe peaches, peeled, stoned and halved
2 tsp freshly squeezed lime juice
100 ml single cream

- Purée the blackberries, reserving 2 for garnish.
- Place the peach halves on dessert plates and drizzle with the lime juice.
- Spoon the blackberry purée into the peaches.
- Top with cream and garnish with the reserved blackberries. Serve immediately.

Carbohydrate content per serving: 20 grams

Tropical fruit salad (FOR 2)

2 kiwi fruit, peeled and sliced
½ a grapefruit, skin removed and chopped into segments
½ a small mango, peeled and chopped
2 tbsp freshly squeezed lemon juice
1 tsp caster sugar
150 ml single cream
Sprigs of fresh mint, to garnish

- Mix together the kiwi fruit, grapefruit, mango, lemon juice and sugar and chill for 30–60 minutes.
- Serve with single cream, garnished with sprigs of mint.

Carbohydrate content per serving: 27 grams

Appendix

Unless otherwise stated, weights are 100 g.

Low-GI Foods

DAIRY PRODUCTS

FOOD ITEM	CARBOHYDRATE (G)	CALORIES
Butter and margarine (15 g)		
Butter (standard)	0	150
Ghee (clarified)	0	150
Margarine	<1	110
Cheese (25 g)		
Brie	<1	91
Camembert	<1	77
Cheddar	<1	100
Cheshire	<1	95
Cottage	<1	25
Cream cheese	<1	84
Edam	<1	88
Emmental	<1	95
Feta	<1	70
Gloucester	<1	100
Goat's cheese	<1	50
Halloumi	<1	60
Lancashire	<1	90
Leicester	<1	100
Mozzarella	<1	75
Parmesan	<1	110
Philadelphia cream cheese	2	70
Ricotta	<1	40
Stilton	<1	92
Wensleydale	<1	92

Prepared cheeses (25 g)

Cheese strings	<1	82
(per stick: 21 g)	<1	69

Cream (100 ml)

Crème fraîche	3	380
Double cream	3	460
Single cream	3	330
Soured cream	4	200

Milk (100 ml)

Cow's milk:		
evaporated	11	160
full-cream	5	66
high-calcium	5	49
semi-skimmed	5	50
skimmed	5	35
UHT longlife	5	68
Goat's milk	4	60
Soya	1	32

DRINKS

FOOD ITEM	CARBOHYDRATE (G)	CALORIES
Coffee (200 ml; decaf)	<1	0
Diet soft drinks (100 ml):		
cola	<1	1
lemonade	<1	3
orange	<1	1
tonic	<1	1
Fruit Shoot (100 ml):		
orange and peach	<1	5
light low-sugar orange	1	8
Sherry (50 ml), dry	2	115
Spirits (25 ml):		
Bacardi	<1	53
brandy	<1	53
gin	<1	53
rum	<1	53
vodka	<1	53
whisky	<1	53
Tea:		
China	<1	0

Sri Lanka	<1	0
Vermouth (50 ml), dry	2	53
Water:		
carbonated	0	0
flavoured (orange)	0	<1
still	0	0
Wine (100 ml):		
red	<1	71
white, dry	<1	75
white, medium	3	77

EGGS

FOOD ITEM	CARBOHYDRATE (G)	CALORIES
Boiled egg	0	147
Duck's egg (large)	0	160
Fried egg	0	147
Omelette	0	147
Poached egg	0	147
Quail's egg	0	15
Scrambled egg	0	147

FISH AND SHELLFISH

FOOD ITEM	CARBOHYDRATE (G)	CALORIES
Fish		
Anchovies (25 g)	<1	45
Bass (25 g)	<1	90
Bream (25 g)	<1	135
Calamari (25 g)	<1	70
Cod :	<1	80
breaded fillet (100 g)	15	200
(per fillet)	20	250
Dover sole (25 g)	<1	80
Haddock:		
fresh (25 g)	<1	100
smoked (25 g)	<1	100
Herring (25 g)	<1	230

Kipper (25 g)	<1	205
Lemon sole (25 g)	<1	95
Mackerel:		
peppered (25 g)	<1	355
smoked (25 g)	<1	190
Salmon:		
fresh (25 g)	<1	200
smoked (25 g)	<1	180
tinned (25 g)	<1	150
Sardines:		
fresh (25 g)	<1	65
tinned (in oil) (25 g)	<1	220
Swordfish (25 g)	<1	120
Trout:		
rainbow (25 g)	<1	125
smoked (25 g)	<1	135
Tuna:		
fresh (25 g)	<1	120
tinned (brine) (25 g)	<1	105
tinned (oil) (25 g)	<1	180
Whiting (25 g)	<1	90
Prepared Fish Products		
Cod fillets (25 g)	<1	76
Fish fingers (100 g)	13	170
(each)	4	50
Shellfish		
Crab:		
fresh (25 g)	<1	120
tinned (25 g)	1	80
Lobster (25 g)	<1	120
Mussels (25 g)	<1	88
Oysters (25 g)	<1	120
Prawns (25 g)	<1	100
Scallops (25 g)	<1	100

HERBS AND SPICES

FOOD ITEM	CARBOHYDRATE (G)	CALORIES
Dried spices (1 tsp) All varieties, including allspice, bay leaf, chilli powder, cinnamon, cloves, cumin, fennel, nutmeg, paprika, pepper, salt and turmeric	<1	10
Fresh herbs (1 tbsp) All varieties, including basil, coriander, dill, lemon grass, mint, oregano, parsley, rosemary and thyme	<1	15–20
Capers	<1	3
Garlic (1 clove)	<1	3
Ginger	7	40
Horseradish	<1	15–20
Rocket (100 g)	2	15
Watercress	2	15–20

MEAT

FOOD ITEM	CARBOHYDRATE (G)	CALORIES
Beef (100 g)		
Beefburgers:		
home-made	0	180
takeaway	20	250
Fillet steak:		
trimmed	0	190
untrimmed	0	210
Kidney	0	150
Liver	0	200
Mince, lean	0	124
Round steak:		
trimmed	0	180
untrimmed	0	200

Rump steak:		
trimmed	0	190
untrimmed	0	270
Sirloin steak:		
trimmed	0	170
untrimmed	0	270
T-bone steak:		
trimmed	0	140
untrimmed	0	170
Topside steak:		
trimmed	0	150
untrimmed	0	170
Lamb, natural		
Cutlet (40 g):		
trimmed	0	90
untrimmed	0	130
Kidney	0	210
Leg (100 g):		
trimmed	0	200
untrimmed	0	220
Liver (100 g)	4	230
Loin chop (50 g):		
trimmed	0	85
untrimmed	0	180
Shank (100 g):		
trimmed	0	140
untrimmed	0	220
Shoulder (100 g)		
trimmed	0	140
untrimmed	0	260
Pork, natural (100 g)		
Bacon	0	260
Fillet	0	170
Leg:		
trimmed	0	170
untrimmed	0	330
Loin chop:		
trimmed	0	170
untrimmed	0	350
Medallion:		
trimmed	0	190
untrimmed	0	300
Mince, lean	0	80
Spare ribs	0	110
Steak:		
trimmed	0	160
untrimmed	0	260

Pork, prepared

Gammon steak (100 g)	0	160
Ham (100 g):		
trimmed	0	100
untrimmed	0	140
Wafer thin	<1	105

OILS, MAYONNAISE AND DRESSINGS

FOOD ITEM	CARBOHYDRATE (G)	CALORIES
Oils		
Corn oil	0	829
Extra-virgin olive oil	0	823
Grapeseed oil	0	829
Groundnut oil	0	829
Olive oil	0	822
Peanut oil	0	899
Sesame oil	0	821
Soya oil	0	899
Sunflower oil	0	828
Virgin olive oil	0	822
Mayonnaise and Vinaigrettes		
Mayonnaise	1	722
Commercial dressings:		
French	15	297
(low-fat French)	9	39
Italian	6	120
(low-fat Italian)	7	32
Vinaigrette, home-made	<1	60
Vinegar (15 ml)		
Balsamic	12	10
Cider	<1	2
Red wine	2	5
Rice	<1	5
White wine	0	5

POULTRY

FOOD ITEM	CARBOHYDRATE (G)	CALORIES
Chicken, natural (100 g)		
Breast:		
skinless	0	170
with skin	0	210
Drumstick:		
skinless	0	90
with skin	0	110
Thigh:		
skinless	0	60
with skin	0	70
Wing:		
skinless	0	70
with skin	0	90
Chicken, prepared (100 g)		
Breast roll	0	120
Drumsticks	0	180
Wings, in barbecue marinade	3	232
Duck (100 g)		
Roast Duck:		
skinless	0	180
with skin	0	300
Turkey, natural (100 g)		
Breast:		
skinless	0	105
with skin	0	140
Mince	0	176
Turkey, prepared (100 g)		
Breast roll	4	92

VEGETABLES AND VEGETABLE PRODUCTS

FOOD ITEM	CARBOHYDRATE (G)	CALORIES
Alfalfa sprouts	4	30
Artichoke:		
globe	1	8
Jerusalem	9	40
Asparagus	1	12
Aubergine	2	14
Beans:		
French	4	25
green	4	25
Beetroot	8	35
Broccoli	1	25
Brussels sprouts	2	25
Cabbage:		
bok choi	<1	12
Chinese	<1	8
red	2	22
savoy	2	20
Carrots	8	37
Cauliflower	2	20
Celeriac	5	30
Celery	3	12
Chilli:		
green	1	20
red	4	26
Courgettes:		
green	2	15
yellow	2	15
Cucumber:		
English	6	9
Lebanese	3	12
Fennel	4	12
Herb salad, commercial	2	15
Leek:		
baby	3	23
standard	3	20
Lettuce:		
cos	2	20
curly endive	2	20
iceberg	2	20
radicchio	2	20
Swiss chard	2	20
Mangetout	5	60
Marrow	4	20

Mushrooms:		
button	2	25
Chinese	15	50
oyster	5	35
Onion:		
brown	4	25
red	4	25
white	4	25
Peas:		
fresh green	6	60
sugar snap	5	33
tinned	9	67
Peppers:		
green	3	15
red	4	25
Radish	2	3
Salad leaves, commercial	2	25
Seaweed	<1	10
Spinach	2	30
Spring onion	4	25
Swede	2	10
Tomato:		
beefsteak	3	20
cherry	3	20
plum	3	20
plum, tinned/peeled	4	24
purée	18	92
round	3	20
vine-ripened	3	20
Turnip	2	12

Commercially prepared vegetables

Sausages, vegetarian:		
organic leek (100 g)	11	195
(per sausage)	5	81
Vegetarian quarter-pounder burgers	7	164

Medium-GI Foods

BREAD, FLOUR AND GRAINS

FOOD ITEM	CARBOHYDRATE (G)	CALORIES
Bread		
Bap (1)	30–41	175–246
Bagel (1)	30	140
Baguette (1)	23	130
Bran loaf (slice)	35	130
Brown bread (slice)	11–20	53–97
Croissant (1)	22	207
Focaccia (1)	30	140
Fruit bread (slice)	15	77
Hamburger roll (1)	40	215
Naan (1)	50	340
Pitta (1)	12–50	55–230
Roll (1)	25–33	150–270
Tortilla (1)	12–25	67–144
White bread (slice)	11–20	50–110
Wholemeal bread (slice)	15–20	77–102
Flour (100 g)		
Corn	90	350
Rice	80	360
Soya:		
(full fat)	23	450
(low fat)	28	350
Wheat:		
plain/white	77	340
self-raising/white	76	330
wholemeal	65	320
Grains (100 g)		
Barley:		
pearl	84	360
wholegrain	65	300
Bulgar	70	330
Couscous	72	355
Oatmeal	70	400
Wheat germ	45	300

DAIRY PRODUCTS

FOOD ITEM	CARBOHYDRATE (G)	CALORIES
Yoghurt (100 ml)		
Acidophilus	8	25
Blackberry and raspberry	15	125
Blackcurrant	17	141
Creamy bio yoghurt	11	130
Natural yoghurt		
full-fat	6	120
Greek	8	100
skimmed-milk	6	50
Raspberry and blackberry		
Strawberry bio yoghurt	9	114
Vanilla flavour/chocolate rice	19	120

DIPS (100 G) AND SNACKS

FOOD ITEM	CARBOHYDRATE (G)	CALORIES
Chilli cheese dip	9	550
Garlic and herb dip	7	370
Hot salsa dip	9	40
Hummus	12	190
Popcorn	71	468

DRINKS

FOOD ITEM	CARBOHYDRATE (G)	CALORIES
Carbonated soft drinks (150 ml)		
cola	16	60
lemonade	16	62
lemon and lime	16	62
Coffee, caffeinated (200 ml)		
black	<1	<1
cappuccino	10	134
white	3	25

Fruit juice (100 ml)
grapefruit (unsweetened)	8	35
lemonade, 'traditional'	18	74
orange, commercial	9	37
orange, fresh	8	33

Wine (100 ml)
rosé	3	75
white, sweet	6	99

FRUIT

FOOD ITEM	CARBOHYDRATE (G)	CALORIES
Apple	10	40
Apricot	7	9
Avocado	2	190
Blackberries (100 g)	12	50
Blueberries (100 g)	13	52
Cherries (100 g)	12	52
Grapefruit	10	51
Grapes (100 g):		
black	15	62
green	12	55
Kiwi fruit	7	35
Lemon	3	11
Lime	<1	8
Melon:		
honeydew (100 g)	6	30
rock (100 g)	5	22
water (100 g)	5	22
Nectarine	7	32
Orange	10	42
Passion fruit	3	20
Peach	8	33
Pear	16	64
Pineapple (100 g)	8	37
Plum	8	34
Raspberries (100 g)	5	24
Rhubarb (100 g)	1	8
Strawberries (100 g)	6	28
Tangerine	7	33

NUTS

FOOD ITEM	CARBOHYDRATE (G)	CALORIES
Almond	7	610
Brazil	3	680
Hazelnut	6	650
Macadamia	5	740
Peanut	12	560
Pecan	6	690
Pine nut	4	690
Pistachio	8	600
Walnut	3	690

PULSES

FOOD ITEM	CARBOHYDRATE (G)	CALORIES
Beans		
Baked beans/tomato sauce	14	75
Black-eye	20	110
Broad	6	150
Butter	12	80
Chickpeas	15	110
Chilli	12	70
Haricot	16	100
Kidney (red)	16	100
Lentils	16	100
Soya:		
bean	5	140
tofu	1	75

SAUCES AND MUSTARDS

FOOD ITEM (100 G)	CARBOHYDRATE (G)	CALORIES
Gravy:		
commercial	10	130
powder	5	25
Pasta sauces, commercial:		
Bolognese	9	52
pesto	60	550
salsa, fresh	8	47
Soy sauce	8	40
Sweet and sour sauce	25	100
Tartare sauce	14	263
Tomato ketchup	25	107
Tomato sauce	35	155
White sauce, home-made	20	200
Worcester sauce	25	110
Mustard		
English	19	190
French	4	104
Wholegrain	4	140

SOUPS (COMMERCIAL)

FOOD ITEM	CARBOHYDRATE (G)	CALORIES
Chicken noodle (100 ml)	5	27
(per serving)	10	54
Cream of chicken (100 ml)	5	51
(per serving)	10	102
Cream of mushroom (100 ml)	5	51
(per serving)	10	102
Cream of tomato (100 ml)	11	71
(per serving)	22	142
French onion (100 ml)	5	25
ʼer serving)	10	50
ʼil (100 ml)	8	41
ʼving)	16	82
ʼɘ (100 ml)	5	30
	10	60
ʼ00 ml)	7	60
	14	120

| Vegetable (100 ml) | 8 | 47 |
| (per serving) | 16 | 94 |

High-GI Foods

BISCUITS, CAKES, PASTRIES AND BUNS

FOOD ITEM	CARBOHYDRATE (G)	CALORIES
Biscuits, sweet (100 g)		
Bourbon	70	500
(per biscuit)	8	60
Chocolate chip	70	500
(per biscuit)	7	50
Cream	70	450
(per biscuit)	7	45
Crunch cream	64	520
(per biscuit)	9	75
Custard cream	65	500
(per biscuit)	8	65
Digestive:		
chocolate	70	500
(per biscuit)	10	75
plain	65	450
(per biscuit)	10	70
Flapjack	57	475
(per biscuit)	13	110
Ginger	80	450
(per biscuit)	8	45
Jaffa cake	70	370
(per biscuit)	10	20
Kit Kat	60	506
(per biscuit)	12	106
Kit Kat Orange	60	506
(per biscuit)	12	106
Rich Tea style	75	460
(per biscuit)	6	35
Shortbread:		
round	65	500
(per slice)	10	80
Scotch finger	70	510
(per piece)	11	90
Shortcake	60	500
(per biscuit)	6	90

Wagon Wheel	68	425
(per biscuit)	27	170

Cakes and Buns (100 g)

Battenberg	50	380
(per slice: 50 g)	25	190
Carrot	45	400
(per slice: 50 g)	23	200
Cheesecake	30	310
(per slice: 50 g)	15	155
Chelsea bun	55	350
(per bun: 75 g)	40	280
Cherry	60	400
(per slice: 50 g)	30	200
Chocolate	60	400
(per slice: 50 g)	30	200
Chocolate éclair	35	380
(per éclair)	25	270
Christmas	60	320
(per slice: 50 g)	30	160
Cream bun	25	425
(per bun: 50 g)	13	210
Crumpet	40	200
(per crumpet)	15	80
Doughnut:		
cream	30	350
iced	45	420
sugar	50	340
Fruit	50	320
(per slice: 50 g)	25	160
Hot cross bun	60	300
(per bun: 50 g)	30	150
Iced fruit bun	45	300
(per bun: 75 g)	33	225
Jam tart	63	390
(per tart: 33 g)	21	130
Lemon curd tart	63	390
(per tart: 33 g)	21	130
Lemon tart	33	415
(per slice: 50 g)	17	208
Madeira	60	400
(per slice: 50 g)	30	200
Marble	60	400
slice: 50 g)	30	200
ffa Cakes	73	398
	5	26

Sponge:		
with jam	60	350
(per slice: 50 g)	30	175
without jam	50	450
(per slice: 50 g)	25	225
Swiss roll	65	350
(per slice: 50 g)	33	175
Viennese cakes	60	500
(per cake: 50 g)	30	250

Crackers and Crispbreads (100 g)		
Cream cracker	65	450
(per cracker)	5	30
Oatcakes	65	450
(per biscuit)	6	45
Rye crispbread	70	330
(per crispbread)	6	25
Water biscuit	80	450
(per biscuit)	5	30
Wholemeal cracker	75	420
(per cracker)	5	30

Pastries (100 g)		
Chocolate	25	300
Croissant	40	350
(per croissant)	25	210
Custard	35	300
Danish:		
apple	45	300
apricot	40	300

CEREALS (100 G)

FOOD ITEM	CARBOHYDRATE (G)	CALORIES
Bran (natural)	60	270
Bran flakes	70	320
Chocolate rice pops	95	380
Coco Pops	85	380
Cornflakes	85	360
Corn Pops	85	380
Crisped rice	90	370
Fibre and fruit flakes	75	350
Fruit and nut flakes	70	350

Honey Loops	77	370
Honey Nut Cheerios	78	372
Honey Puffs	90	390
Muesli	70	360
Oats, instant	70	370
Porridge oats	73	400
Sugar-coated cornflakes	90	370
Sugar puffed wheat	85	350
Sultana bran flakes	20	300

CONFECTIONERY

FOOD ITEM	CARBOHYDRATE (G)	CALORIES
Chocolate		
Bounty	56	485
Cooking	60	500
Double Decker	65	460
Flake	55	530
Fruit and nut	55	550
Fudge	72	445
Maltesers	61	490
Mars Bar	70	450
Milk	60	520
Milky Way	72	454
Mini Eggs	68	495
(per egg)	2	15
Orange	57	530
Ripple	59	528
Yorkie bar	58	526
Sweets		
Chewing gum:		
normal – with sugar	30	100
(per piece)	3	10
sugar-free	<1	40
(per piece)	<1	4
Fudge	80	450
Liquorice	65	280
Cherry sherbet sweets	93	380

CRISPS AND SNACKS

FOOD ITEM	CARBOHYDRATE (G)	CALORIES
Bombay mix (100 g)	34	544
Dipping chips (100 g)	63	490
Potato crisps		
Cheese and onion (100 g)	48	535
(per bag)	12	134
Potato sticks (100 g)	52	530
(per bag)	39	400
Prawn cocktail (100 g)	49	535
(per bag)	12	134
Prawn crackers (100 g)	60	534
Pringles Original (100 g)	48	544
Roast beef (100 g)	47	540
(per bag)	12	136
Roast chicken (100 g)	46	550
(per bag)	12	140
Salt and vinegar (100 g)	45	550
(per bag)	11	140
Sour cream and onion (100 g)	65	435
(per bag)	14	94
Tomato (100 g)	45	550
(per bag)	12	140

DESSERTS

FOOD ITEM	CARBOHYDRATE (G)	CALORIES
Apple pie	30	200
Chocolate mousse	30	225
Chocolate sponge pudding	40	210
Christmas pudding	60	340
Creamed rice	17	100
Crème caramel	20	120
Custard:		
pouring	15	90
powder/full-cream milk	12	100
Ice cream, vanilla	24	190
Lemon meringue pie	40	320
Lemon mousse	20	185
(light)	20	140

Raspberry mousse	30	245
Strawberry and cream sundae	17	236
Strawberry cream trifle	22	170
Strawberry trifle	18	150
Trifle	30	100

DRINKS

FOOD ITEM	CARBOHYDRATE (G)	CALORIES
Beer (pint):		
ale	16–30	165–320
bitter	14	190
stout	10	200
Cider (pint):		
dry	15	205
sweet	25	240
Milkshakes, thick (100 ml):		
chocolate	20	120
strawberry	20	120
Port (50 ml)	6	75
Sherry (50 ml):		
medium	3	60
sweet	4	70

FAST FOOD

FOOD ITEM	CARBOHYDRATE (G)	CALORIES
Bacon and egg muffin (100 g)	25	250
(per muffin)	33	380
Big Mac	44	490
Cheeseburger (100 g)	30	250
(per burger)	33	300
Chicken dippers (100 g)	13	280
(per dipper)	2	50
Chicken, fried (100 g)	25	230
(per piece, approx.)	45	420
Chicken McNuggets (per 6)	12	250
(per nugget)	2	42

Chicken nuggets (100 g)	15	125
(per nugget)	3	24
Chips:		
fried (100 g)	30	190
oven (100 g)	30	160
takeaway (100 g)	30	240
French fries:		
oven-bake (100 g)	36	240
(per portion)	28	220
takeaway (100 g)	34	280
Hamburger, takeaway (per burger)	33	250
Hash brown (100 g)	30	230
(per piece)	15	120
McChicken Sandwich		
(per sandwich)	38	375
Onion bhaji (100 g)	16	300
(per bhaji)	4	65
Pizza (all varieties high GI):		
average pizza (100 g)	33	250
(per slice)	25	170
cheese and tomato,		
deep pan (100 g)	45	310
(per slice)	45	310
cheese and tomato,		
thin and crispy (100 g)	28	260
(per slice)	25	230
four cheese,		
thin and crispy (100 g)	32	250
(per slice)	20	155
pepperoni (100 g)	32	267
(per slice)	20	164
vegetable and goat's		
cheese,		
thin and crispy (100 g)	31	250
(per slice)	21	165
Quarter-pounder (100 g)	20	240
(per burger)	37	420
Saffron rice (100 g)	24	155
Sausage roll (100 g)	25	300
(per roll)	30	370
Spring roll (100 g)	25	230
(per roll)	50	400
Vegetable pakora (100 g)	20	265
(per pakora)	5	60
Vegetable samosa (100 g)	25	225
(per samosa)	7	60

FRUIT

FOOD ITEM	CARBOHYDRATE (G)	CALORIES
Banana	31	125
Mango	20	80

JAMS AND MARMALADES (100 G)

FOOD ITEM	CARBOHYDRATE (G)	CALORIES
Jam:		
fruit	69	260
low sugar	32	123
Marmalade	69	260

NUTS

FOOD ITEM	CARBOHYDRATE (G)	CALORIES
Cashew	18	570
Chestnuts	36	170

PASTA AND NOODLES

FOOD ITEM	CARBOHYDRATE (G)	CALORIES
Commercial pasta products (100 g)		
Macaroni cheese	15	120
Ravioli in tomato sauce	13	73
Spaghetti hoops	12	56
Spaghetti in tomato sauce	13	61
Noodles (100 g dry weight)		
Egg noodles	70	340

Pasta (100 g dry weight)
All varieties including cannelloni,
conchiglioni, farfalle, fettuccine,
fusilli, gnocchi, lasagne, linguine,
pappardelle, penne, rigatoni,
spaghetti, tagliatelle and vermicelli · 73 · 360

RICE (DRY WEIGHT)

FOOD ITEM	CARBOHYDRATE (G)	CALORIES
Arborio	78	350
Basmati	76	350
Brown	74	349
Thai fragrant	77	350
White rice:		
long-grain	76	340
short-grain	78	375
wholegrain	75	350

SAUCES AND STOCKS

FOOD ITEM	CARBOHYDRATE (G)	CALORIES
Sauces		
Barbecue	65	270
Chilli	50	50
Chutney	55	200
Hoisin	38	180
Horseradish	10	105
HP	27	119
Mango chutney	58	230
Oyster	35	190
Satay	35	450
Seafood	20	335
Commercial stocks		
Bisto:		
chicken gravy granules	56	389
original	55	390
vegetarian granules	55	394

Knorr stock cubes:

beef	21	326
chicken	24	301
lamb	16	295
vegetable	22	308

OXO stock cubes:

beef	38	265
chicken	37	243
lamb	43	289
vegetable	42	253

SUGAR

Caster	100	400
Demerara	100	394
Granulated	100	400
Icing	100	398

VEGETABLES

FOOD ITEM	CARBOHYDRATE (G)	CALORIES
Mushrooms, shiitake, dried	64	295
Parsnip	14	65
Potato	16	75
Sweet potato	20	80

Index